What People A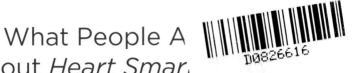 About *Heart Smar*

"We have been advocates for women's health for many years. Our goal is to ensure that all women are familiar with the fact that heart disease is different in women. Women should have access to the knowledge, the services and the tools to live long, healthy lives. *Heart Smart for Women* is an important resource for women of all ages who want to take the journey to living a more heart-healthy life. With real-life, practical advice on everything from nutrition information to sleep habits and stress management to finding a true physician partner, *Heart Smart for Women* teaches women how to be proactive about their health, and take the small steps that will have a huge impact on their heart health."

—Iris and Saul Katz

"Self-management and patient/provider partnerships are pivotal for the heart health of women. Drs. Mieres and Rosen have provided women the impetus, resources and skill sets for this momentous undertaking!"

—Nanette K. Wenger, MD
Professor of Medicine (Cardiology) Emeritus,
Emory University School of Medicine and
Founding Consultant, Emory Women's Heart Center

"*Heart Smart for Women* is a must read for women as well as their health care professionals. The book provides a roadmap for simple lifestyle changes that, as physicians, we should all be recommending to the women in our care. It is an armamentarium for members of the health care community who want to ensure that their female patients are living the most heart-healthy life possible. An added benefit is that because women are the drivers of overall family health, women following the six-week program will likely make their entire families healthier."

— **Lawrence Smith, MD**
 Founding Dean
 Donald and Barbara Zucker School of Medicine at Hofstra/Northwell

"The most comprehensive lifestyle plan for optimal heart health tailored to the unique needs of women that I have read. This book offers a straightforward and easy-to-follow approach for creating a healthy lifestyle, reducing stress, improving your diet and exercising effectively. Importantly, this book is written by leading authorities in the field of cardiovascular prevention and women's health. This book stands above all others as the book to have and to use as a guide to make important and positive heart-healthy changes in your life."

— **Leslee Shaw, PhD**
 Professor of Medicine,
 Emory University School of Medicine

"As a pediatric cardiologist, I know that heart disease in women has very early roots – from family risk factors to dietary habits and lifestyle choices. Drs. Mieres and Rosen provide clear guidance on the important steps that women of all ages can take to insure a heart healthy future. If an ounce of prevention is worth a pound of cure, then women who read this wonderful book will quickly realize that it is worth its weight in gold."

— **Angela Romano, MD**
 Pediatric Cardiologist,
 Cohen Children's Medical Center, Northwell Health

"Thirteen years ago, I experienced a rare form of heart attack. My successful recovery was due to two brilliant and dedicated women cardiologists – Dr. Stacey Rosen and Dr. Jennifer Mieres. They each partnered with me and played an important role, guiding and teaching me how to live a heart-healthy life, all of which is now captured in this wonderful book, *Heart Smart for Women*. Their real and commonsense suggestions, their thoughtfulness and their way of just simply encouraging and LOVING me brought me to my happy place. I now pay it forward, inspired and mentored by Drs. Rosen and Mieres, as a WomenHeart Champion, facilitating a support group for women living with or at risk of heart disease."

— **Joyce Lenard, WomenHeart Champion**

"Heart Smart for Women is a guide made for every woman. Dr. Jennifer Mieres and Dr. Stacey Rosen have developed a Six S.T.E.P.S. in Six Weeks Program that will help you understand if you are at risk for heart disease and empower you to take control of your own heart health. This book is the first step to improve the dialogue between women and their physicians, with the goal of identifying risk factors for heart disease, reducing heart disease and ultimately saving more women's lives."

— **Martha Gulati, MD**
   Chief of Cardiology, University of Arizona
   Editor-in Chief, *CardioSmart*
   Author of *Saving Women's Hearts*

"Heart Smart for Women is a must-read for all women who want a healthy heart. The information from two experienced cardiologists outlines easy-to-follow steps we all can take to optimize our heart health in six weeks. The book comes complete with questions for your doctor, exercises, food lists and portion sizes. Be smart and read this book for optimum health."

— **Robin Miller, MD, MHS**
   Co-Author of *The Smart Woman's Guide to Midlife and Beyond* **and**
   Healed: Health and Wellness for the 21st Century

"Heart disease is the #1 cause of death for women and still too few women know this. Heart disease in women is under-diagnosed and under-treated. All women should read *Heart Smart for Women*; it will empower them to understand and reduce their risk of heart disease. Everything you do that is good for your heart is good for the rest of you. Dr. Jennifer Mieres and Dr. Stacey Rosen, world class experts, share their knowledge in a straightforward and engaging way. Buy one for you and buy one for a woman you love."

—**Holly S. Andersen, MD**
The Ronald O. Perelman Heart Institute
The New York Presbyterian Hospital

"This book should be required reading for all women who want to live a long and healthy life. The information presented offers women knowledge and encouragement to protect and preserve their heart health. Women who follow the simple steps outlined here will be forever grateful. Give a copy to every woman you love!"

— **Susan M. Campbell, MPH**
Vice President of Public Policy, WomenHeart

"Prevention of cardiac events is a struggle that I have lived with for many years. *Heart Smart for Women* contains so much information, from the explanation of heart disease to tests to real patient accounts, and that's only the first half! Everyone can learn something from the six steps. It's in easy, understandable terms that explain the "how to" part of managing and living with heart disease. This book is wonderful!"

— **Portia Rindos, RN**

"*Heart Smart for Women* is a meticulously-researched and beautifully written guide to achieving heart health. It champions a unique program that promotes life-long healthy choices using techniques that every woman can embrace, regardless of age."

— **Penny Stern, MD, MPH**
  Director, Preventive Medicine, Northwell Health

"*Heart Smart for Women* is the GPS for women to most efficiently optimize their heart health and that of their families and communities."

— **C. Noel Bairey Merz, MD**
  Director, Barbra Streisand Women's Heart Center
  Professor of Medicine, Cedars-Sinai Medical Center

Heart Smart
FOR
Women

To Linda,

Heart Smart
FOR
Women

SIX S.T.E.P.S. IN SIX WEEKS
TO HEART-HEALTHY LIVING

Jennifer H. Mieres, MD, FACC
Stacey E. Rosen, MD, FACC

with Sotiria Everett, EdD, RD and Lori M. Russo, JD

Stay Heart Smart!!

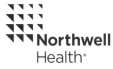

Northwell
Health®
Katz Institute for Women's Health

Copyright © 2017 by Jennifer H. Mieres, Stacey E. Rosen

All rights reserved.

This book or any portion thereof may not be reproduced or used in any manner whatsoever without the express written permission of the authors except for the use of brief quotations in a book review.

This book is for informational purposes only and is not intended to take the place of medical advice from a trained medical professional. You are advised to consult a doctor or qualified health professional before acting on any of the information in this book.

Printed in the United States of America

First Printing, 2017

ISBN 978-0-9849005-4-1

Onward Publishing, Inc.
464 Main Street
Port Jefferson, NY 11777
www.onwardpublishing.com

To all of the strong women in our lives who have partnered with us on this journey, from whom we continue to learn each and every day.

Table of Contents

Foreword

As a woman, a physician and the daughter of a cardiologist, I recognize the importance of heart disease prevention and awareness... especially for women. There is an urgent need for better communication of critical information, and no one does this better than Drs. Mieres and Rosen et al. There are many good books on this topic, but this one truly could save your life.

Consider this: Though heart disease is the leading cause of death in women, statistics show that only 17 percent of women know that it is their greatest personal health risk. Heart disease in women is under-diagnosed and under-researched, so it's significant to receive such conclusive medical insight from Drs. Mieres and Rosen, leading cardiologists with over 50 years of combined experience in cardiovascular medicine.

One of the reasons that some ignore personal health is because it demands a change that can at times be daunting. Another reason is that we simply don't understand how our bodies work nor where we should start with lifestyle changes. *Heart Smart for Women* helps us navigate through an evidence-based blueprint for personal implementation and rules out any reluctance we might have on how to begin this journey. This book is a well-rounded resource that demystifies the science, biology and statistics about our bodies and translates its meaning into clear, simple steps that make changing habits doable.

Let's be honest, ladies, knowledge is key, but what's more important is that we move into action! There are solutions that can help us achieve the level of wellness we all desire. The great thing is that this can be an exciting journey! Let this book be the turning point to making your health a priority. Find the courage to take the steps needed toward heart-healthy living and do it the "heart smart" way!

Jennifer Ashton, MD, MS, FACOG, Ob-Gyn,
ABC News Chief Women's Health Correspondent

Introduction

We have all heard the adage, "If you have your health, you have everything." This bit of timeless wisdom often gets lost in or pushed aside by demands of our busy lives. Yet without good health, everything else pales.

Good health is not a given. It is something we must work for by taking control of our lives and putting ourselves first. Yet women often put themselves last, considering the needs of their family and friends above their own. We want to help you break this cycle and place you firmly on the road to living a heart-healthy life.

We each have more than 25 years of medical experience in the field of cardiology, and we share a passion for educating and empowering women to be active participants and effective advocates for their health.

This book is a call to action for women everywhere. The message is a positive one: Heart disease is preventable! More than 90 percent of all women have one or more risk factors of heart disease, and more than 44 million women living in the United States – about a third of the female population – suffer from some form of heart disease. However, every one has the opportunity to conquer it and live well. In fact, research has shown that women can lower their risk of heart disease by as much as 80 percent simply by making healthy lifestyle changes. This can be anything from choosing to move every day to decreasing the amount of unhealthy fats in your daily diet. Any type of daily exercise, combined with small but meaningful changes in your daily food choices, can have a tremendous impact on your health.

Awareness. Simple lifestyle changes. Forming a true partnership with your doctor. These are the key elements of heart health. Yet these elements so often elude us. We think we are too busy, too set in our ways, too old or too young to form new habits and learn new approaches to preventing, minimizing or reversing heart disease. But recent advances in the medical and scientific communities demonstrate that the opposite is true: it is never too soon or too late to adopt heart-healthy habits. Behaviors become habits in just three weeks. So if you follow our Six S.T.E.P.S. in Six Weeks to Heart-Healthy Living Program, by the end of those six weeks, the new behaviors you have learned will have become habits. And these habits will put you well on your way to living a heart-healthy life.

Heart disease is an equal opportunity killer, and so this book is for all women, from all walks of life, of all ages and all ethnicities. Heart disease continues to be the leading cause of death of women in the United States (lung cancer is the second-leading cause of death). Heart Disease claims more lives than breast cancer, more lives than all cancers combined. But the amazing fact is that over 80 percent of all heart disease is preventable! Great strides have been made in the prevention, early diagnosis and treatment of heart disease in women. But awareness of these facts is not enough. Knowledge must be translated into action, and without simple lifestyle changes and doctor-patient partnerships, these strides will not translate into actual lives saved.

We have met many women with heart disease or risk factors for heart disease who are eager to make heart-smart changes in their lives but don't know how to begin. Our mission is to demystify the science, the biology and the statistics surrounding heart disease, and to provide concrete, simple steps to begin the journey.

Heart Smart for Women will help you understand the science behind heart disease. It also provides simple lifestyle changes you can make in your approach to eating, cooking and exercising and offers concrete suggestions on how to develop the most effective partnership with your doctor. All of these things will help you eliminate this potential killer from your life and improve the quality of your daily living.

We want you to continue to enjoy the foods you love, but we have highlighted simple changes to recipes, ingredients and portion sizes that will yield a healthier version of those foods. You will find ways to maintain control of what you eat when dining out as well as when dining at home. You will also learn ways to incorporate exercise into your daily routine, even if you are convinced that you don't have an extra minute in your already jam-packed day.

We know our program works because we have seen the proof again and again with our patients. We guarantee that with our six-week program you'll be on your way to living a heart-healthy life – moving more, eating better, living with less stress and savoring life more.

This book was inspired by the thousands of incredible women we have met as patients and at community lectures and health screenings over the past 25 years. It is meant to empower you and to translate the knowledge of heart disease into an action plan that will put you firmly on the road to heart-healthy living.

Jennifer H. Mieres, MD, FACC, FAHA

Stacey E. Rosen, MD, FACC, FAHA

Overview

The more you know about heart disease and the simple but critical steps you can take to reduce your personal risk of developing heart disease, the more successful you will be on your journey to heart health. Toward that end, this book is separated into two parts:

Part One provides a comprehensive discussion of the workings of the healthy heart and the risk factors, signs and symptoms of heart disease. We hope you find it enlightening! You may want to refer back to Part One as needed. The important thing is that you familiarize yourself with the vocabulary of heart disease so that you can comfortably communicate with your doctor and better advocate for your own health care.

Part One will help you identify and assess your own risk factors for developing heart disease so that you understand the special issues you may face. It will also provide the necessary background regarding the "whys" of the Six S.T.E.P.S. in Six Weeks to Heart-Healthy Living Program and how they may apply to your particular health situation.

Part Two provides the "how," with the complete Six S.T.E.P.S. in Six Weeks to Heart-Healthy Living Program. Here you will find a week-by-week roadmap for your journey to heart health, including choosing the right foods, dining at home and out of the home, finding a doctor who is the right physician-partner for you and learning to maximize sleep and minimize stress.

Important note to the reader: This book is for informational purposes only and is not intended to take the place of medical advice from a trained medical professional. You are advised to consult a doctor or qualified health professional before acting on any of the information in this book.

Part One

Women and Heart Disease:
An Overview

"I think it is important for every woman
to decide to be healthy, to be wise and
to be kind."

– Maya Angelou

Understanding Heart Disease in Women

We are fortunate to live at a time when great strides are being made toward the better understanding of heart disease and how it affects both men and women. We know now that heart disease is an equal opportunity killer, and the number one cause of death of women in the United States. However, just over half of American women identify it as such and only 17 percent see it as a personal threat. During the past two decades the medical and scientific communities have gained tremendous insights into some of the unique health risks of women, and significant progress has been made toward reducing the number of women with heart disease. Yet every day there are women of varying backgrounds and ages whose stories tell us that there is much work to be done; women who remind us that we must all be vigilant about our own health, and that the way to address our own risks of developing heart disease is to make simple lifestyle changes and establish a true partnership with our health care providers.

We want to introduce you to some of the women in our community. Their stories are different, their backgrounds diverse, yet they all have one important similarity.

Claudia is a 48-year-old Caucasian woman whose high-pressure job at a bank and busy family life keep her in a constant state of anxiety. She is often tired, experiences occasional heart palpitations and sometimes feels as if she can't breathe.

Chandra is a 29-year-old graduate student of South Asian descent, with a beautiful newborn baby girl. Chandra had an easy, uneventful pregnancy until she reached week 24, when her blood pressure skyrocketed.

Theresa is a 35-year-old Latina who works as an assistant to the president of a small department store. Theresa has a history of elevated blood sugar and was recently diagnosed with Type 2 diabetes.

Sasha is a 59-year-old Black woman who is trained as a physical therapist but now spends her days caring for her elderly mother at home. Recently, she has had several bouts of severe indigestion and nausea, and an overwhelming cold and clammy feeling. She is sure she is coming down with flu.

Rebecca is a 42-year-old woman of Puerto Rican descent who is a nurse on a cardiac unit of a large hospital. She has been extremely fatigued lately although her schedule has not changed.

These five women represent different walks of life, age brackets and ethnicities, yet they are the same in one important respect. They all have signs and risk factors of heart disease.

We will follow two of these women more closely as we learn about their challenges and triumphs on their journeys to heart-smart living.

Let's begin with the story of Claudia, who works as a vice president at one of the country's leading banks. Claudia has a busy and full life. Since her promotion to VP five years ago, her daily work routine has been stressful, requiring long hours and frequent travel. In addition, her home life is quite active, as she and her husband have two teenage daughters with busy school and sports schedules of their own.

Claudia is very disciplined. She understands the importance of exercise and is careful to adhere to a daily exercise routine of a 30-minute aerobic workout five days a week, combined with two days of strength training with light weights. But over the past two months, Claudia has noticed a change in her energy level. She is fatigued after only 15 minutes on the treadmill. On weekends, while running her usual errands, she is dragging. She has begun making small changes to her routine to compensate, such as parking her car right next to the store entrance to minimize the walking distance.

At first, Claudia assumed that her fatigue was a normal byproduct of perimenopause; however, as the months went by, her low energy and fatigue continued. She has noticed something else – something that is definitely out of character for her. Last month, during a particularly stressful period at work, she lost her temper with a colleague who was only doing his job in delivering some upsetting financial news. This colleague was only the messenger! Claudia was confused by her own behavior, as she has always prided herself on her ability to remain calm under pressure. In addition, she has experienced episodes of palpitations and a feeling of anxiety leading to left upper back pain. Fortunately, it is time for Claudia's annual checkup.

What Is Heart Disease?

Heart disease, which is also sometimes referred to as cardiovascular disease (CVD), is an umbrella term that includes a range of diseases of the heart and blood vessels. The primary culprit of heart disease is atherosclerosis, the process whereby plaque, made up of substances that circulate in your blood including calcium, fat and cholesterol, builds up in the blood vessels, leading to the thickening and narrowing of the vessel walls. The buildup of plaque in the blood vessels that supply the heart can lead to a heart attack. Although heart disease is the focus of this book, our program is designed to prevent and control the risks for all conditions caused by atherosclerosis, which include heart attack and stroke. We mention heart attack and stroke together because your risk factors for heart disease also increase your chances of having a stroke. As you follow the program you will not only be improving your heart and the vessels that supply it, but also be positively affecting the blood vessels that supply your brain.

The Unique Challenge of Heart Disease

The fact that women are far more likely to die of heart disease than from all forms of cancer – in fact, from all other diseases – combined is a clear indication of how important it is to know how to prevent or stop it. This can sometimes be difficult because heart disease can masquerade as indigestion and delay early diagnosis. Remember:

- Heart disease is hard to diagnose in its early stages.

- Heart disease has no outward manifestation to announce its presence and get us to seek treatment.

- Heart disease can build up over years, or sometimes decades, until it makes itself known (for many women that means since their twenties!) often in the form of a heart attack or stroke.

But it does not have to be that way. Heart disease is preventable and treatable – and, as we go through the steps to heart health together, you will learn how to keep this most important organ healthy.

Know the Facts

To get a clear understanding of where heart disease ranks in terms of women's health, here's a quick look at the numbers.

According to the American Heart Association:

- **Nine out of 10** women have one or more risk factors for heart disease,

- **One in three** women will die of heart disease,

  but

- **One in eight** women will develop breast cancer, and

- **One in 26** women will die of breast cancer.

In addition, as highlighted by the Framingham Heart Study, a study of the health of the residents of Framingham, Massachusetts, that has been ongoing since 1948, a diabetic woman is three to seven times more likely to have heart disease than a diabetic man.

These are remarkable statistics for a disease that has historically been considered a "man's disease." There have been numerous national awareness campaigns about women and heart disease, but recent surveys have demonstrated that lack of awareness remains a problem across all races. Only two-thirds of white women are aware that heart disease is the leading cause of death, and only one-third of Black and Hispanic women and one-tenth of South Asian women recognize the threat that heart disease poses to their health.

The Causes of Heart Disease: Men vs. Women

Heart disease, as we said earlier, is an equal opportunity killer. What that means is that *women and men are at equal risk of developing heart disease and suffering a heart attack.* In fact, until 2013, more women died each year from heart disease than men! However, when it comes to the prevention, diagnosis and treatment of heart disease, until recently, most research and treatments have been focused on men. The medical and scientific communities have historically underestimated the prevalence and importance of heart disease in women. For many years, this resulted in a failure to study the differences in the way men and women develop and experience heart disease. In fact, it is only within the past two decades that the medical and scientific communities expanded their research focus to include all aspects of women's heart health, from risk factors to diagnosis to treatment.

There are certain risk factors that men and women share. These include: smoking, high blood pressure (hypertension), diabetes, sedentary lifestyle, high cholesterol and family history of heart problems. The more risk factors you have, regardless of whether you are a man or a woman, the greater your chances of having a heart attack or stroke. But there are important differences that are unique to and can be more dangerous for women:

- Women typically develop heart problems about seven to 10 years later in life than men do, but by about the age of 65 men and women suffer from heart disease at the same rate.

- Diabetes is a much more potent risk factor for women than for men. Diabetic women are three to seven times more likely to die from heart disease than diabetic men.

- Women tend to be more obese, more inclined to have a sedentary lifestyle and more likely to suffer from hypertension and diabetes than men.

- Certain conditions play a much more important role leading to heart disease and heart attacks in women. These include: lupus or rheumatoid arthritis and other inflammatory or autoimmune disorders, obstructive sleep apnea, radiation-induced heart disease, stress, depression and anxiety.

- Women with pregnancy-related complications of gestational diabetes, hypertension, preeclampsia, eclampsia and preterm delivery are at increased risk for heart disease five to 15 years after delivery.

- Women with early-onset menopause (i.e., before age 40) are at greater risk than other women due to an early loss of estrogen, which is cardioprotective.

The Added Risk for Women of Black, Latina or South Asian Heritage

In addition to the risk factors for women mentioned above, Black women, Latina women and women of South Asian descent have an even higher risk of heart disease than Caucasian women – as much as a 69 percent higher risk – due to their higher incidence of high blood pressure, obesity, physical inactivity, diabetes and metabolic syndrome (a group of risk factors that includes increased amounts of abdominal fat, high blood pressure, high cholesterol levels and insulin resistance or glucose intolerance). Studies show that these risk factors can be more potent and prevalent in these ethnic groups.

What Does This Mean to Your Heart Health as a Woman?

Knowledge Is Power

Now you know the statistics and can see how many women are affected by heart disease. But we want to stress a point we made earlier: *More than 80 percent of heart disease is preventable!* Our goal is to give you the added knowledge you need to clearly understand the science behind heart disease and then enable you to make simple lifestyle changes to prevent or stop the development of this disease. You can continue to enjoy your traditional foods, but now you will have information on how to prepare meals in healthier ways. Some of you may have to lose a few pounds, but even for those of you who don't, learning to control portion size is key not only to controlling your weight but also to keeping blood sugar and cholesterol levels within range. Moreover, you will learn that it is possible to reach and maintain a healthy weight *without depriving yourself* or going on a severely restrictive diet. We will also suggest how you can make simple changes to your daily routine to become more active. You'll be delighted and surprised at how these easy changes add up and ultimately lead to the major improvements necessary to keep yourself healthy.

One goal of the Six S.T.E.P.S. in Six Weeks Program is for you to share what you learn with your family and friends, thereby improving their health and ultimately helping to break the cycle of heart disease. *Prevention* is key, and a whopping 80-plus percent of heart disease can be prevented through *early recognition* of symptoms, accurate *diagnosis* and *treatment*. In addition, *simple lifestyle changes* make a huge impact in reducing risk.

For some of us, heart disease starts as early as our twenties and continues silently, slowly blocking the arteries with plaque buildup. Heart disease, as we now know, is different not only between women and men, but also among women of different races.

So turn the page and get started as you discover how getting and staying healthy can be so much easier and more fun than you had ever imagined. Experience first-hand how following our program over the next six weeks can put you on a lifelong road to good health. We promise that you will feel better, look better and have more energy while reversing the path of heart disease.

As cardiologists, we have over 50 years of combined experience in cardiovascular medicine, treating women of all races, ethnicities and ages. Our program works, and we have thousands of success stories to prove it. But before you begin the Six S.T.E.P.S. in Six Weeks Program, it is important that you understand more about your heart, and how it works.

The Healthy Heart vs. the Diseased Heart

Throughout human history, the beat of the human heart has signified life. The heart itself not only is the symbol for love but through the ages has also been considered the organ closest to the soul. The ancients believed what we now know to be true: The heart is the most important organ in the body.

Now we would like to explain how your heart works, what happens when it doesn't and what the conditions are that lead to heart disease. This knowledge will help you put to use what you'll learn later in the book about keeping this organ healthy.

Although some of the information presented is fairly technical, please bear with us. It's important that you be familiar with the structure and workings of your heart along with the causes of problems. Use this chapter as a resource and refer back to it from time to time, because what might not make perfect sense now *will* later on as you build your heart knowledge and vocabulary. Now, let's learn anatomy!

The Healthy Heart – a Very Efficient Pump

This first lesson in anatomy illustrates not only how the heart is constructed but how and why a healthy heart functions the way it does. Once you understand what the physical heart looks like inside and out, you will be able to envision how this hard-working organ goes about its job pumping life-giving blood through the body. You will also be able to visualize what actually happens to this amazing muscle when things go wrong.

The healthy heart is a simple and efficient fist-sized pump that sits in the center of your chest and beats approximately 72 times per minute, which is roughly 100,000 times every day. The heart's primary job is to pump nutrient-rich blood to all of the body's vital organs through a large set of tubes called arteries. Over the course of an average lifetime (approximately 81 years for women) the heart will beat more than three billion times without ever resting. Here's how it does it.

Heart Anatomy

Two Sides/Four Chambers/Four Valves

The heart is divided into two sides, separated by a wall called the septum. Each side has an upper and lower chamber, which are separated by structures called valves. The valves work like one-way doors that open to allow blood to flow through to the next chamber but close so the blood cannot flow backward. (It's the valves opening and closing that make the "lub-dub" sound, but more about this later.)

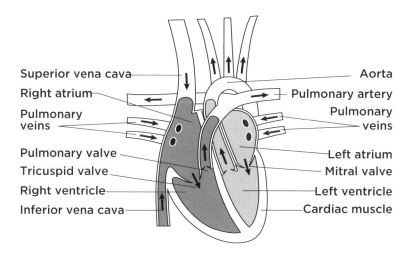

The anatomy of the heart.

The right side of the heart (the left side in the illustration) pumps blood *to* the lungs where it gets oxygen.

The left side of the heart (the right side in the illustration) *receives* the oxygen-rich blood and pumps it throughout the body.

The atria are the upper two chambers. They collect blood flowing *into* the heart.

The ventricles are the lower two chambers. They pump blood *out* of the heart.

The tricuspid valve separates the right atrium and right ventricle.

The pulmonary valve separates the right ventricle and the pulmonary artery, which carries the blood *to* the lungs.

The mitral valve separates the left atrium and the left ventricle.

The aortic valve separates the left ventricle and the aorta, which pumps blood *through* the body.

Arteries and Veins

The arteries and veins are the major blood vessels that get blood to and from the heart and deliver blood throughout the body.

The pulmonary artery carries blood to the lungs to pick up oxygen.

The aorta is the body's main artery and carries oxygen-rich blood to the body.

The pulmonary veins bring oxygen-rich blood from the lungs to the heart.

The superior and inferior vena cava are large veins that return the blood from the body back to the heart.

The coronary arteries get oxygen-rich blood from the aorta to the heart itself, which needs its own supply of blood to function.

How the Heart Works

To give you a better idea of exactly how this miraculous pump works, let's follow the blood on its journey through the circulatory system.

Starting on the right side…

In search of oxygen, blood comes into the heart through the *superior and inferior vena cava* where it fills the *right atrium.*

The right atrium then contracts to open the *tricuspid valve* to allow this blood to move down into the *right ventricle*.

When the right ventricle is full, the tricuspid valve closes and the ventricle contracts to open the *pulmonary valve* so the blood can travel through the right and left *pulmonary arteries* to each lung for oxygen.

Returning on the left side...

This oxygenated blood then returns to the heart through the right and left *pulmonary veins* where it fills the *left atrium*. The left atrium contracts to open the *mitral valve* and allow the blood to move into the *left ventricle.*

When the left ventricle is full, the mitral valve closes and the ventricle contracts to open the *aortic valve* so the oxygen-rich blood can travel into the *aorta* and throughout the body. But just beyond the aortic valve are the *left and right coronary arteries* that will detour some of this oxygen-rich blood to nourish the heart itself.

The Sound of Your Heartbeat

As we mentioned, the "lub-dub" sound that your doctor hears through the stethoscope is made when the heart valves open and close. It happens like this:

The "lub" sound comes from the closing of the mitral and tricuspid valves when the ventricles contract to pump blood out of the heart. The "dub" sound comes from the closing of the aortic and pulmonary valves when the ventricles relax to fill with blood from the atria.

Cardiac murmurs are extra sounds in between the "lub" and the "dub" that are heard with a stethoscope. Some may be related to normal flow of blood and are often called innocent or benign murmurs. But others may represent a range of heart abnormalities. If your health care professional detects a cardiac murmur, he or she will let you know if additional evaluation is recommended.

Your Heart's Electrical System

Along with the heart chambers, valves and blood vessels, the heart contains a sophisticated electrical system that produces the "spark" to drive the pumping of the heart. The heart contains an internal pacemaker and electrical circuits that allow it to work consistently over a lifetime.

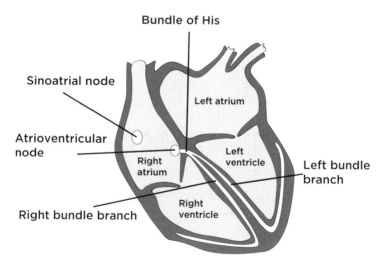

The normal heartbeat begins when the sinoatrial node produces an electrical signal. This electrical signal travels first through the two atria and then through the two ventricles via specialized wiring in the atria and the ventricles.

Taking Care of Your Amazing Heart

This wondrous organ is designed to work long and hard, but in order for it to do its job, it must be taken care of properly. If any of the mechanical components get damaged or the blood vessels get clogged, then the heart cannot function as it should. So let's take a look at what happens when problems do occur.

The Diseased Heart: What's Happening?

Heart disease is a general term used to describe a range of diseases that affect the heart and blood vessels. It can be related to the heart itself (a heart attack, heart failure, an electrical disorder); to the brain (a stroke); or to the blood vessels or circulatory systems that supply other critical organs (like the kidneys or extremities).

Conditions Related to the Heart

Heart attack is the most common type of heart problem that occurs when the coronary arteries (the blood vessels that wrap around the surface of the heart and supply it with blood) are blocked enough to deprive the heart muscle of the blood it needs to function. If blood supply is limited for too long, the heart muscle will not recover, and this leads to formation of a scar in part of the left ventricle. This is commonly related to coronary artery disease (CAD), which is due to blockages in the coronary arteries that can limit blood flow.

Ischemia is the medical term describing an insufficient blood supply to nourish the organs of the body. In the case of ischemic heart disease, inadequate blood supply to the heart muscle usually leads to symptoms such as shortness of breath, lightheadedness, chest pain or pressure (called angina), pain in the left arm or left shoulder, jaw or throat as well as heartburn or feelings of general fatigue. These symptoms can worsen during any type of exertion (exercise, climbing stairs, housework, etc.) or during times of emotional stress. Sometimes, however, this lack of adequate blood supply does not give rise to symptoms; that is, it can be "silent." Silent ischemia is said to occur when evidence of heart damage is found in the absence of the symptoms described above.

Ischemic heart disease is a relatively new term often used today to describe the full range of coronary heart disease (CHD).

Coronary artery disease happens when there is plaque buildup inside the main or smaller coronary arteries. This can lead to a reduction in blood supply, which could cause a heart attack. This condition is called *atherosclerosis* – commonly known as hardening of the arteries. The heart muscle needs oxygen in order to function, and the coronary arteries are the pipes through which the blood transports that oxygen to the heart – like the pipes that transport water in your home. It's important that they remain open.

Recently, scientists have discovered that heart attacks can occur in the absence of atherosclerosis. Other abnormalities of blood vessels can also lead to heart attack. These include vessel spasm, or *microvascular dysfunction*, a new term describing blood vessels that do not dilate normally during stress or exercise, which can lead to insufficient blood flow to the heart. These abnormalities can lead to the same types of symptoms and can cause heart muscle damage but without any blockages in the arteries.

Spontaneous Coronary Artery Dissection, also known as SCAD, is an emergency condition that occurs when a tear forms in the wall of a coronary artery. As blood flow is slowed or blocked entirely, the result can be a heart attack, heart rhythm abnormalities, or sudden death. The causes of SCAD are still uncertain. However, the condition, which occurs more often in women than in men, is considered rare. It typically impacts women between the ages of 30 and 50 with no prior history of or risk factors for heart disease. SCAD can occur during pregnancy or in the first few weeks after delivery.

Because SCAD results in ischemia, symptoms of SCAD are consistent with those of other forms of ischemic heart disease.

Takotsubo cardiomyopathy, also known as "broken heart syndrome " or stress cardiomyopathy, is a temporary condition that occurs as a result of acute weakening of the left ventricle, usually related to severe emotional or physical stress. The exact cause is not known, but experts think that surging stress hormones "stun" the heart, and trigger changes in the heart muscle cells or coronary blood vessels (or both) that prevent the left ventricle from pumping effectively. Takotsubo cardiomyopathy occurs mainly in women and presents in the same way as a classic heart attack. Symptoms include chest pain and shortness of breath after severe physical or emotional stress and are often indistinguishable from those of a heart attack. The good news is that, once diagnosed and treated, it is usually reversible, and rarely recurs.

Arrhythmia describes an abnormal heart rhythm, or a heart-beat that is too slow, too fast or irregular. Any irregular heartbeat will affect how efficiently the heart is working and how well blood is being pumped throughout the body.

If an arrhythmia is brief, it is experienced as a skipped heartbeat and is generally nothing to be concerned about. However, a severe arrhythmia can result in significant and long-lasting palpitations, lightheadedness, fainting or even death.

Heart failure is a misleading term, because the heart doesn't actually fail. Think of it more as damage that results in the heart being unable to effectively pump blood to the entire body. The inability to pump efficiently leads to fluid buildup in the lungs and other tissues with symptoms that include fatigue, shortness of breath, loss of appetite, nausea and swollen feet and ankles. Heart failure is more common in women over the age of 60 and is often related to an under-lying problem such as heart attack, high blood pressure, diabetes or heart valve problems. Each year, more than one million women in the U.S. will develop heart failure. There is also a form of heart failure that younger women may develop during or shortly after pregnancy, called *peripartum cardiomyopathy*.

We now know that there is a form of heart failure where the heart pumps effectively but is less able to relax to allow blood to flow into the ventricles. This is called *heart failure with preserved ejection fraction (HFpEF)*. HFpEF is a more com-mon form of heart failure in women than in men and has been found to be challenging to diagnose and treat. Approx-imately 61 to 76 percent of patients with HFpEF are women. Current research is focused on better ways to diagnose and treat this form of heart failure. Nonischemic heart failure is more common in women than in men. This makes sense because diabetes, hypertension and obesity are more prevalent in women and are also stronger risk factors in women than in men.

Valvular heart disease occurs when there is an abnormality of any of the four heart valves that separate the chambers of the heart; one (or more) of the valves doesn't open enough to allow blood to flow freely (stenosis) or doesn't close tightly enough to prevent blood from flowing backward (regurgitation). Stenosis and/or regurgitation can develop in any of the four valves, but both are more common on the left side of the heart involving the aortic or mitral valves. Certain forms of valve disease are related to advanced age, but others may be related to infections or other conditions.

Conditions Related to the Brain

Stroke (cerebrovascular accident) is to the brain what a heart attack is to the heart, and it usually happens for the same reason: when blood flow is blocked or interrupted. When any part of the brain is deprived of nutrient-rich blood, irreversible damage can be the result. This is why, as with symptoms of heart attack, it is important to get stroke victims treated as soon as possible. Symptoms of a stroke include speech abnormalities, facial drooping and arm or leg weakness.

Conditions Related to the Circulatory System

Deep vein thrombosis is a serious condition where blood clots form in the veins, usually in the leg. These clots can dislodge, travel through the bloodstream to an artery in a lung and block blood flow, resulting in a condition called *pulmonary embolism* (see below).

Pulmonary embolism is a sudden blockage in an artery going to the lung caused by a blood clot that was formed someplace else in the body. This blood clot is capable of causing permanent damage to the lung, and this can prevent other organs from getting the oxygenated blood they need to function. A pulmonary embolism can lead to heart failure or death, whether caused by one large clot or many smaller clots.

Hypertensive heart disease refers to heart damage that results from high blood pressure (hypertension); it may lead to coronary artery disease, heart failure and thickening of the heart muscle.

Hypertension is a dangerous disease because it causes no symptoms but can lead to heart attack, heart failure, stroke or kidney failure. Hypertension can be treated and kept under control with regular checkups and medication. Hypertension is more prevalent in post-menopausal women.

Peripheral artery disease (PAD) is a disease in the arteries far from the heart. PAD results from atherosclerosis (the formation of fatty deposits in the blood vessels), which prevents sufficient flow of blood to the kidneys, arms, legs and feet. Its consequences can be anything from cramping of the legs, either when walking or resting, to permanent damage to these body parts if blood is severely restricted. If the kidneys are involved, chronic kidney disease or kidney failure can be the result. People with PAD are also at a very high risk of having a stroke or a heart attack.

Important Risk Factors for Heart Disease

Ischemic heart disease (CHD) is the most common form of heart disease; it begins with damage to the lining and inner layers of the coronary arteries. The following risk factors have been shown to increase your chances of suffering damage to these arteries. We have separated these risks factors into three categories: nonmodifiable risk factors, modifiable risk factors (including those that can be treated to lessen the risk) and modifiable risk factors that are more potent for or unique to women.

Nonmodifiable Risk Factors:

- Heredity (including family history, race and ethnicity)
- Age
- Gender

Modifiable Risk Factors:

- Smoking, including secondhand smoke
- High blood pressure (hypertension)
- Abnormal blood sugar (diabetes or prediabetes)
- Elevated cholesterol (hyperlipidemia)
- Sedentary lifestyle
- Being overweight or obese

Modifiable Risk Factors That Are More Potent for or Unique to Women:

- Pregnancy-related hypertension (eclampsia or pre-eclampsia) or abnormalities of sugar (gestational diabetes)

- Autoimmune disease such as lupus or rheumatoid arthritis

- Depression, anxiety and other psychosocial risk factors

Other Contributing Factors:

- Stress

- Insufficient sleep

- Alcohol abuse

- Poor diet and nutrition

Surprisingly, damage to the lining of the arteries can begin as early as young adulthood and lead to the buildup of plaque in the coronary arteries that continues throughout adulthood. Over time, this plaque can slowly grow to narrow or completely obstruct the artery, resulting in the chest pain or discomfort that we call angina. In the case of a nonobstructing plaque, the plaque can acutely rupture, leading to a heart attack. This is called a *vulnerable plaque*. Even if it doesn't rupture, this hardened plaque builds up inside the coronary arteries, causing them to narrow, and this reduces the flow of oxygen-rich blood to the heart muscle.

Now that you understand the key features of the heart and how disease affects how the heart works, let's turn our attention to how best to prevent and control these risk factors so you can live free of coronary heart disease. As you read on, you'll find the tools you need to identify your personal risk of developing CHD, minimize the impact those risk factors may have on your life and start your journey to living a heart-smart life!

Assessing Your Risk for Heart Disease

Even though heart disease is very serious, *it is largely preventable and treatable*. Each day, you have the opportunity to make choices that will protect you from the likelihood of developing heart disease. Women from all walks of life have learned how to make healthy, permanent changes to their lives in order to prevent heart disease or lessen its impact.

Rebecca

In Chapter 1, we introduced you to Rebecca, a 42-year-old Latina woman. We now want to share with you more of Rebecca's story and her journey to heart-healthy living.

For 20 years Rebecca worked as a nurse on the cardiac service at a large hospital. But one day she found herself in the waiting room of the imaging center of that hospital, not as a nurse but as a patient scheduled for a stress test. As she waited for her name to be called, she reflected on the sequence of events that led her here.

It had all started the previous month, when she began feeling fatigued and had difficulty catching her breath when she climbed stairs or walked quickly when food shopping. For the past three years she had been going through the stress of a divorce after finding out her husband had been unfaithful. Now that her divorce was finalized, she was finally feeling optimistic about the future. But Rebecca didn't know how to slow down and take it easy. She typically worked four 10-hour shifts each week, with most of that time spent on her feet. In addition, she had a busy domestic life with two teenagers at home – a son in high school and a daughter in community college – and she also cared for her increasingly disabled mother. Rebecca often found herself unable to get a good night's sleep.

Ironically, Rebecca's job as a nurse was to care for women and men recovering from heart attacks, yet not for one moment did she consider that her own symptoms of fatigue and shortness of breath were warning signs of heart disease. She reasoned that she had no chest pain and she was still able to do her job, so her symptoms could not possibly mean that she had heart disease.

In the waiting room, nervously waiting to be called in for her stress test, she distracted herself by picking up a brochure that described the symptoms of heart disease in women and how they can differ from the typical male symptoms. What she read made the hairs on the back of her neck stand up. She realized that she, a health care professional, didn't even know that the warning signs of heart disease in women might be different from those in men!

Rebecca thought about her constant exhaustion and recalled those occasions when she experienced mild upper back pain – usually when climbing stairs – that she ignored or attributed to a number of excuses: weight gain, lack of regular physical activity, the stress related to her divorce and being a single mom and caregiver.

But as she continued to read, she began to acknowledge the fact that she had many of the risk factors for heart disease, including:

- Early menopause (age 40)

- Treatment for mild hypertension

- Slow but steady weight gain to nearly obese (15 pounds, mostly stored around a 39-inch waist)

- High body mass index (BMI) of 29

In addition, Rebecca recalled that the bloodwork done at her yearly visit to her internist six months ago showed she was prediabetic and at risk for diabetes, and her blood pressure was high. At that time, her doctor had put her on an anti-hypertensive medication and reassured her that if she made some changes to her diet and decreased her waist circumference, she would be in good shape. They agreed to revisit this at her next appointment.

Rebecca had the classic signs, but she hadn't put them together, and initially, neither had her doctor. And here she was, scheduled for a stress test only because of the urging of a worried colleague.

One week earlier, at the end of a 10-hour shift, Rebecca had experienced left upper back pain. She felt extremely fatigued and was short of breath. Her colleague noticed her sitting and resting before being able to head home and convinced her to speak to the cardiologist on call that night. The cardiologist wisely suggested that she be evaluated to find out why she was feeling this way.

As she sat in the waiting room, knowing what she now knew, Rebecca was concerned. She was keeping her fingers crossed that she would be fine.

Rebecca's wakeup call came just in time. Her stress test revealed that she didn't have significant ischemic heart disease; her symptoms were caused by poorly controlled hypertension. In fact, her blood pressure at the end of her stress test was markedly elevated, at 210/110. She realized that, while she was taking the blood pressure medication prescribed by her doctor, she had never followed up with him to check to be sure that it was effective and that the dosage was correct.

At her follow-up visit a few days later, her cardiologist customized the same Six S.T.E.P.S. in Six Weeks Program you will find in Part Two of this book. Rebecca's progress was impressive. By her next visit to her cardiologist she had lost seven pounds and one inch off her waist, her blood pressure was within normal range at 118/78, she was sleeping better and she had more energy.

The Sobering Statistics

Below is a recap of some of the important statistics presented in Chapter 1:

- Between 1984 and 2012, cardiovascular disease (including heart disease and stroke) killed more women than men. Since then, the rates are basically the same.

- One woman dies every 80 seconds from cardiovascular disease.

- One in every three deaths of women each year is caused by cardiovascular disease.

- 90 percent of women have one or more risk factors for cardiovascular disease.

- Fewer women survive their first heart attack than men.

- Certain risk factors for heart disease are more potent for Black, Latina and South Asian women.

The Good News

We know from the findings of the American Heart Association (AHA), through their Go Red for Women movement, that:

- 80 percent of heart disease is preventable through lifestyle changes and education.

- Women who participate in heart-healthy programs actually do reap the benefits they promise by adopting healthier habits.

- Over the past 10 years the death rate of women from heart disease has decreased more than 30 percent, which translates to 670,000 women's lives saved.

These encouraging statistics are the direct result of an increased understanding on the part of the medical community about how women present with heart disease as well as the healthy behavioral changes women have made. These changes include such things as: losing weight, increasing exercise, making healthy diet changes, keeping track of cholesterol, blood sugar and blood pressure levels and partnering with their doctors to learn how to start a heart-healthy plan. Taking an active role in your health will help you feel better and live longer.

Make It Personal: Take Stock of Your Risk Factors

When it comes to risk factors for heart disease, the science is clear: The sooner you identify and address your risk factors, the less likely you are to develop heart disease and the healthier you will be. We hope you'll take the following, literally, to heart.

Although women generally have the same heart disease risk factors as men, there are some risk factors that either affect women exclusively, such as pregnancy-related issues and issues surrounding menopause, or affect women differently, for example, diabetes, which raises the risk of heart disease more in women than in men. What is common to both sexes is that our risk for heart disease and heart attack rises with the number of risk factors each of us has as well as the severity of each of those risk factors. What's more, risk factors tend to "snowball" and worsen each other's effects. This means that having one risk factor doubles your risk for heart disease, having two risk factors increases your chance for heart disease fourfold and having three or more risk factors increases your risk for heart disease more than tenfold. Complicating this snowball effect is that some risk factors are worse than others. For example, smoking and diabetes put you at far greater risk for heart disease and heart attack than other risk factors.

It is important to remember that:

- More than 75 percent of women ages 40 to 60 (the menopausal years) have one or more risk factors for heart disease. It is during these years that forming a partnership with your doctor is of critical importance, and identifying your risk factors and adopting a healthier lifestyle can have a significant impact in decreasing your risk for heart disease.

• Women also are at greater risk than men when it comes to having heart disease or a stroke, especially if they are Black, Latina or of South Asian descent.

But there is a way to significantly improve those odds by making simple lifestyle changes. For example, sustained moderate exercise can significantly decrease your chance of heart disease by positively impacting several risk factors, such as lowering blood pressure, improving cholesterol profile and achieving a healthy weight.

Identify, Address and Modify Your Risk Factors

The goal of this book is to empower you to identify, address and modify the factors that put you at risk for heart disease. As medical professionals, we fully recognize that some of the most potent risk factors are the most difficult to address. Quitting smoking, losing weight, managing stress and becoming more active may seem overwhelming at first. But we will offer you suggestions, advice and tips on how to start the journey toward living a more heart-smart life. This is not an all-or-nothing proposition! Each small change can make a difference and have a big impact on your heart health.

If you haven't identified a primary care physician who understands issues related to women's heart health, you will find suggestions in Week 4 of the Six S.T.E.P.S. in Six Weeks

Program on how to choose a doctor with whom you can partner. If you are already seeing a doctor or are taking medications for other risk factors, then be sure to follow your doctor's instructions regarding lifestyle choices and take your medication exactly as prescribed. Don't be shy about asking questions if there is something you don't understand. If you're diabetic, be diligent about checking your blood sugar and keeping your numbers in the normal range. There are dozens of small decisions we make each day that give us the opportunity to improve our heart health and minimize our chances of ever having a heart attack.

Create a *Personal Health Inventory*

As a first step on your journey to heart health, you will need an accurate inventory of your overall health. Keeping this inventory will be one of the biggest assets in your quest to stay heart healthy. Just as a physician or nurse makes notes in your chart when you come in for an office visit, you need to do the same for yourself. This is the start of your journal – which we call your *Personal Health Inventory*. Keeping track of all the details about your personal health in one document will be a real eye-opener. This information will help you keep track of the things you want to discus with your doctor and serve as a foundation to allow you and your doctor to customize an overall health plan. It also will be a way to have all of your health information at your fingertips, including your family medical history, your personal medical history (all surgeries, medical procedures, hospitalizations, pregnancy-related issues, etc.), allergies, the medications or supplements you currently take and their dosage (including any reactions or side effects experienced from other medications you have previously taken), your insurance numbers, your doctor's instructions and your treatment plan.

A journal can take whatever form you prefer. It will be a constantly evolving record, and it will be important to keep it up to date. Some people like to use a fancy notebook, while others use an electronic tablet or smartphone, a legal pad, even a three-ring binder. Whatever works best for you is all that matters, but if you opt for keeping a digital journal, be sure to secure and protect all data appropriately and optimize privacy settings.

Keeping a *Personal Health Inventory* is easy once you begin. Later we will provide details on how to approach this. **But to start, your *Personal Health Inventory* should include a listing of all of your risk factors, starting with:**

Risk Factors You Cannot Change (Nonmodifiable)

Your Family History and Genetics

The most important risk factor that we cannot change is our family history. We are all products of our family's genetic makeup, and our risk of heart disease is greatly impacted by our genetic composition. Think of your family members, take stock of their health and make a list of any medical issues they have. Start with your immediate family. For example, do you have a male parent or sibling, living or dead, who had a heart attack or stroke or suffered from heart disease at age 55 or younger, or a female parent or sibling who had the same at age 65 or younger? **If so, write down his or her relationship**

to you and as detailed a description as you can provide of the nature of his/her heart condition.

Having parents or siblings with early heart disease increases your risk, too. Your *Personal Health Inventory* will show you if you are at risk through heredity. Discussing your family history of heart disease accurately with your doctor is an excellent first step to early identification, proper screening and treatment for you.

Even though a family history of heart disease significantly increases your risk, knowing about it can make all the difference in your own health. Once you are aware that you may be at high risk, you have the information that will allow you to make changes.

It is useful to note in your *Personal Health Inventory* other important health conditions of your immediate family.

Race and Ethnicity

The past two decades of medical and scientific research have shown us the importance of studying heart disease in a gender-, race- and ethnicity-specific way. Just as we learned that heart disease in women can be different from heart disease in men, we have also learned that Black, Latina and South Asian women may be affected by risk factors differently than Caucasian women. Black and Hispanic women are generally at higher risk due to the prevalence and potency of such risk factors as high blood pressure, diabetes, physical inactivity and challenges with maintaining a healthy weight. Women of South Asian descent are more likely to have abnormal cholesterol and triglycerides and prediabetes profiles, which in turn increase the likelihood of having heart disease.

Simply being aware of these additional risks and how they are influenced by your heritage will give you a head start in warding off potential health problems or treating current ones.

Our goal is to educate women from all walks of life so that you can narrow the odds of developing heart disease and learn about the additional health problems that some of us carry in our genes. Because of genetic factors, you might be at higher risk than someone in another racial or ethnic group, but the playing field is leveled when it comes to environmental factors – if you know what to do. The key is prevention, and the Six S.T.E.P.S. in Six Weeks Program is designed to help you get there.

Note your race and ethnic background in your *Personal Health Inventory* so that you can discuss with your physician whether your race or ethnicity brings with it any additional risks or requires any special precautions on your road to heart health.

Age

The risk of developing heart disease increases with age. In addition, post-menopausal women are at greater risk than premenopausal women. **So, make a note of your present age in your *Personal Health Inventory* and, if applicable, the age you went through menopause.**

Risk Factors You Can Modify (Modifiable)

Diabetes (High Blood Sugar) and Prediabetes

Diabetes is a disease in which the body's blood sugar level is too high. This is because the body doesn't make enough insulin (generally referred to as Type 1 diabetes) or does make insulin but doesn't process it effectively (generally referred to as Type 2 diabetes). Insulin is a hormone that helps move blood sugar into cells where it's used for energy. Over time, a high blood sugar level is dangerous because it contributes to increased plaque buildup in the arteries. Diabetes and prediabetes raise the risk of heart disease more in women than in men, and having diabetes can almost double a woman's risk of developing heart disease. Prediabetes is a condition in which the blood sugar level is higher than normal, but not as high as with diabetes. However, prediabetes also puts you at higher risk for developing both diabetes and heart disease.

Before menopause, estrogen provides women some protection against heart disease, but women who are diabetic lose the protective effects of estrogen. Diabetes is a major risk factor for heart disease because the body needs help in controlling blood sugar through diet, medication, insulin or a combination of the three. Uncontrolled diabetes is a particularly worrisome risk factor for women but becomes even more dangerous for women who have other, simultaneous risk factors such as high cholesterol, hypertension or obesity.

If you have diabetes, prediabetes or insulin resistance, add this fact to your *Personal Health Inventory*.

If you have diabetes, it is very important that you check your blood regularly, make smart food choices, maintain an ideal body weight and exercise regularly. If you are taking medication or using insulin, use as directed. People who learn to manage their diabetes can live long, healthy and active lives.

The blood test to diagnose diabetes and prediabetes is the hemoglobin A1c (HbA1c). It provides clinicians with an accurate picture of what a person's average blood sugar levels have been over a period of weeks/months.

Normal HbA1c:	under 5.7 percent
Prediabetes:	5.7 to 6.4 percent
Diabetes:	6.5 percent or above confirmed on two separate occasions

Recently, the medical community recommended that this test be the primary test used to diagnose all forms of diabetes, as opposed to the fasting blood glucose test of years past.

Hypertension (High Blood Pressure)

Blood pressure is the measured force of the blood against the artery walls. This pressure is recorded in two numbers. The higher number is the systolic pressure, which represents the pressure in the arteries when the heart is pumping blood, and the lower number is the diastolic pressure, which represents the pressure in the arteries when the heart muscle is relaxing (i.e., between heartbeats). The following chart reflects the categories established by the American Heart Association with respect to hypertension.

Blood Pressure Category	Systolic Blood Pressure (mmHg)		Diastolic Blood Pressure (mmHg)
Normal	Under 120	and	under 80
Prehypertension	120 to 139	or	80 to 89
Hypertension Stage 1	140 to 159	or	90 to 99
Hypertension Stage 2	160 or higher	or	100 or higher

When a person has high blood pressure, the heart muscle works harder than it should, which can lead to atherosclerosis. There are no real symptoms of high blood pressure, so if you haven't visited your doctor in some time you may not know that you have it. It is very important to have it checked regularly. According to the American Heart Association, one in four women has high blood pressure, and 60 percent of those don't know they have it – which is why hypertension is called the silent killer!

Again, we want you to think about your relatives, since high blood pressure often runs in families. **Make a note of any who suffer from it in your *Personal Health Inventory.*** Additionally, high blood pressure often affects women who are overweight and/or eat a diet high in salt. **If you have been diagnosed with high blood pressure, including gestational hypertension (even if it resolved after giving birth), note that as well.**

The rate of high blood pressure in women over the age of 20 is 46 percent for Black women and 30 percent for Latina and Caucasian women. Over the age of 50, all women are twice as likely as men to have hypertension. But again, hypertension can be controlled with medication, salt restriction, weight control and regular exercise.

Lipids (LDL and HDL Cholesterol and Triglycerides)

There has been considerable controversy recently relating to the impact of cholesterol on our health. Explaining cholesterol can be confusing, but we can simplify it. Cholesterol is a soft, fatlike substance found in the cells of the body and circulating in the blood. If you have too much cholesterol, it interacts with other substances to form plaque in the lining of the arteries, causing atherosclerosis.

Cholesterol travels in the bloodstream in small packages called lipoproteins. The two major kinds of lipoproteins are *low-density-lipoprotein (LDL)* cholesterol and *high-density-lipoprotein (HDL)* cholesterol. LDL cholesterol is sometimes called "bad" cholesterol because it carries cholesterol to tissues, including heart arteries, while HDL cholesterol is sometimes called "good" cholesterol because it helps remove cholesterol from the heart arteries.

A blood test called a lipoprotein panel is used to measure cholesterol levels. This test gives information about total cholesterol, LDL cholesterol, HDL cholesterol and triglycerides, another type of fat found in the blood, which we will discuss on the next page.

Cholesterol levels are measured in milligrams (mg) of cholesterol per deciliter (dL) of blood. An abnormal cholesterol panel is generally defined as total cholesterol of greater than 200 mg/dL, with an LDL cholesterol level greater than 100 mg/dL, and/or an HDL cholesterol level less than 50 mg/dL.

In addition to cholesterol, there are *triglycerides*, which represent the most common type of fat in the body. Too much presents a powerful risk factor for women. We now know that a woman's HDL cholesterol and triglyceride levels predict her risk for CHD better than her total cholesterol or LDL cholesterol levels. A triglyceride level greater than or equal to 150 mg/dL is considered elevated. Recently the American Heart Association and the American College of Cardiology have created a more personalized approach to identifying your risk for heart disease, called the ASCVD (AtheroSclerotic CardioVascular Disease) Risk Estimator. Women who have not previously had a heart attack or stroke can use this tool. It uses your information (including race, gender, age, cholesterol numbers and blood pressure) to calculate your risk of heart disease. You can find the ASCVD tool at www.tools.acc.org.

If you have or an immediate family member has high cholesterol or triglyceride levels, please note this in your *Personal Health Inventory*.

Again, exercise and a healthy diet low in sugar and saturated fats help decrease cholesterol levels. There is also evidence that cholesterol-lowering medications, called statins, can reduce the incidence of heart disease and heart attack for women.

Overweight/Obesity

People who are overweight have a greater chance of also having high blood pressure, diabetes and elevated cholesterol levels. An overweight or obese woman is three times more likely to have heart disease than a woman of normal body weight for her height. Being overweight is a very common problem today among all women, as are the health issues it creates. **If you fall into the overweight or obese category, mark it in your *Personal Health Inventory*.**

The interesting thing about weight loss is that, for many, just losing as little as five to eight pounds can help to get blood pressure under control, improve blood sugar and decrease lipid levels, thereby lowering the risk of developing heart disease or having a heart attack. Slow and steady weight loss is recommended, as opposed to what is sometimes called "yo-yo" dieting or "weight cycling," where weight is lost and gained quickly and repeatedly. A recent study of post-menopausal women suggests that women whose weight goes up and down dramatically are at increased risk for heart disease.

What's important for women to understand is the fact that it's not just how much extra weight they carry, but *where* they carry it. Women who carry much of their fat around the waist are referred to as apple-shaped and are at highest risk for heart disease. Women who carry most of their fat on their hips and thighs are referred to as pear-shaped and are at lower risk for heart disease than those who are apple-shaped.

To get the full picture of how excess weight affects your risk, you need to know your body mass index (BMI) and waist measurement. The BMI is the measure of an individual's body fat based on her weight in relation to her height. If you have a BMI greater than 24.9 and a waist measurement greater than 35 inches, you're at increased risk. If your waist measurement divided by your hip measurement is greater than 0.9, you're also at increased risk. You can determine your BMI by visiting the National Heart and Lung Institute website: www.nhlbi.nih.gov.

Metabolic Syndrome

The term *metabolic syndrome* refers to a group of risk factors that tend to occur together. This includes low HDL, high triglycerides, elevated blood pressure, abnormal blood sugar and abdominal obesity. A diagnosis of metabolic syndrome is made if you have three of these five risk factors.

Cigarette Smoking/Secondhand Smoke

Not only does smoking increase the risk of having heart disease and a heart attack, but it is the leading preventable cause of heart disease. Just in case you need a little more persuading: Women smokers are six times more likely to have coronary artery disease than nonsmokers. Smoking has a negative impact on cholesterol levels, as there is evidence that it encourages blood platelets to clump within coronary arteries, making a heart attack more likely. Smoking also has an impact on microvascular dysfunction, leading to blood vessels that do not behave normally, with resulting angina and heart attack (see Chapter 2).

Smoking only a few cigarettes a day can *double* your risk of coronary artery disease as compared to a nonsmoker, and we're not even mentioning lung cancer, COPD, macular degeneration and a host of other problems that smoking complicates, such as diabetes and high blood pressure. The good news is that when you quit smoking, that risk starts decreasing immediately, and over time the risk goes away.

Exposure to secondhand smoke increases the risk of heart disease in the same way. So ask your smoking friends and relatives to step outside if they want to smoke and you want to stay healthy.

If you still smoke or live in a household where smoking is tolerated, then note that in your *Personal Health Inventory* and work with your housemates or family members to develop a plan to create a smoke-free living environment.

Recently, some people have tried to cut back on their cigarette smoking by turning to e-cigarettes. However, clinical studies on the effects of e-cigarettes suggest that toxic effects of nicotine in traditional cigarettes also exist with e-cigarettes. At this time, we do not recommend the use of e-cigarettes as a tool to stop smoking.

There is no way to sugar-coat this message: Smoking kills. There are many new medications and quitting aids on the market (with and without a prescription) that can help you kick the habit. Schedule a visit with your doctor and discuss the best way to stop. You can also get help by calling the National Cancer Institute's Smoking Quit Line (1-877-44U-QUIT) for advice provided by their trained personnel, or by contacting your local hospital or health system; many have smoking cessation programs for community members. With the current price of cigarettes, quitting will also save you money. So, quit today and start saving for that vacation, that special dress or that show you've been wanting to see. What a great way to celebrate your new, healthier lifestyle.

Lack of Physical Activity

We're not saying you need to join a gym, but we are saying that to keep your heart healthy, you must maintain an active lifestyle. Changes as minor as adding a brisk walk for 30 minutes each day (three 10-minute walks have the same benefit), taking the stairs instead of the elevator or parking your car at the far end of the shopping center lot all contribute to a more active you! The advice is simple: We all need to "choose to move" more. An inactive lifestyle leads to a higher incidence of high blood pressure, obesity and elevated cholesterol.

You may have heard the term *exercise-related cardioprotection.* This refers to the fact that physical activity leads to improvement in many of the risk factors described previously. Active women have a significantly decreased incidence of heart disease. **If you are not moving around as much as you should, add this risk factor to your *Personal Health Inventory.*** Remember, too, that any movement is good. This includes cleaning the house, walking the dog, running around after the kids or grandkids, dancing, bicycling, etc. Thirty to 45 minutes of activity three times a week is all you need for a healthy heart and a more fit you.

 A wearable tracking device can be useful for counting your steps as well as reminding you to get up and walk around if you have been sitting for longer than one hour. Read more about these devices in Week 2 of our Six S.T.E.P.S. in Six Weeks Program.

Stress

Stress is something we must all learn to live with, but too much stress takes its toll on our heart health. How we react to stress varies from person to person, but most of us could benefit from finding creative ways to make our lives less stressful. We've all been there – some things may roll off our backs today but send us into a tailspin tomorrow. And we all have friends who seem to manage stress beautifully, while others simply do not.

There are also different types of stress. Events over which we have no control may wreak havoc on our lives when we least expect it, but sometimes we experience stress that we have created ourselves.

Here's an example: If you are the type of person who leaves everything to the last minute, you may then experience anxiety trying to meet a deadline or be on time. But you can implement some time-management lifestyle changes to make your life run more smoothly. Or maybe you stress out and feel guilty about taking time out for yourself to relax. But having no down time takes its toll on your health. **So if you are feeling stressed for any reason, make a note of it in your *Personal Health Inventory* along with your reasons for feeling this way.**

Learning how to manage stress is important for overall health as well as heart health. Take a look at your daily routine, including your personal, family and work relationships, with an eye to lessening stress.

Sleep

We know for certain that not getting enough sleep can set you up for heart problems. Without adequate sleep the body simply cannot function as it should. Our circadian rhythm (a cycle of approximately 24 hours) tells our bodies when to sleep, rise and eat. If you don't have regular sleep habits or don't get enough sleep, your body's functions will not be in balance. When you stay awake for too long you are fighting the body's natural tendency to rest, and that can be harmful to your overall health.

Chronically disrupted or insufficient sleep can affect everything from your critical thinking ability to your mental health and sex drive. Lack of sleep may actually even increase your risk of death from all causes. If you rely on taking medication to control important health issues like high blood pressure, then the efficacy of the medications may be lessened by poor sleep habits.

The bottom line is that your body needs rest to recharge itself, to keep the immune system in peak condition and to keep your circadian rhythm in its normal cycle. We all need enough sleep to ensure that we stay healthy and safe, make sound decisions and can adequately deal with the stresses and challenges of daily life.

Seven hours of sleep every night is the minimum amount of sleep we need. Sleep time cannot be "made up" on weekends! **If you are unable to get enough sleep, note it in your *Personal Health Inventory*; it can be an important clue if you develop health issues, start forgetting things or just don't feel like yourself.**

Getting adequate rest is one of the most important things you can do for your overall health and well-being. A well-rested person is alert, has the energy needed to exercise, looks great and is better able to fight off illness.

Risk Factors That Are More Potent for or Unique To Women

Autoimmune Diseases

Recent research shows that in women the presence of autoimmune diseases such as lupus and rheumatoid arthritis has been linked to a higher risk of atherosclerosis, which as you will recall from Chapter 2 is the buildup of plaque and fat in the arteries. Plaque buildup in the coronary arteries can lead to blockages in blood flow to the heart, which can result in heart attack. Women suffer from autoimmune diseases at a significantly higher rate than men. If you suffer from an autoimmune disease such as lupus or rheumatoid arthritis and have other risk factors for heart disease, you are at greater risk for developing heart disease at a younger age. This autoimmune condition also inhibits the natural protection of estrogen in premenopausal women.

The human body's immune system functions as a complex network of special cells and organs designed to defend the body against germs and other foreign invaders. At its core your immune system has the unique ability to identify your own tissues and distinguish them from foreign invaders like bacteria or viruses. But sometimes a flaw develops that hinders its ability to make this distinction, and the body starts producing autoantibodies that attack normal cells by mistake. Special cells called regulatory T cells, whose job it is to keep the immune system in line, also fail. The end result is a misguided attack on the body by itself.

What parts of the body are affected depends on which of the 80 known types of autoimmune diseases is at work. Although there is no cure for these autoimmune diseases, treatment options have been continually improving. In addition to medications, a healthy weight, physical activity and sufficient sleep have all been shown to have a positive effect on symptoms. **Autoimmune diseases seem to run in families, so be sure to include information in your *Personal Health Inventory* about any family members with any of these conditions.**

Rheumatoid Arthritis

Rheumatoid arthritis, also known as RA, is the most common type of autoimmune disease and is more common among women than men. It tends to strike women at younger ages than men, and women tend to respond less well to treatment. The disease attacks the lining of the joints throughout the body, making them painful, stiff, swollen and deformed.

Systemic Lupus Erythematosus

Systemic lupus erythematosus, also known as SLE or lupus, is the most common type of lupus and the type of the disease that attacks connective tissue. It mainly affects women, but men do get it. Lupus can produce painful and swollen joints as well as harm the heart, kidneys, skin, lungs and other organs. The disease does not have a predictable course; women with lupus are subject to flare-ups followed by remission.

Some signs of lupus are:

- "Butterfly" rash across the nose and cheeks

- Rashes on other parts of the body

- Painful or swollen joints and muscle pain

- Hair loss

- Headaches and severe fatigue

Sjögren's Syndrome

Sjogren's (SHOH-grins) syndrome is a disorder of the immune system that targets the glands that make moisture. Its most common symptoms are dry eyes and dry mouth. Sjogren's syndrome is often seen in those who have other immune system disorders such as rheumatoid arthritis and lupus. Women are affected more often than men, and it is more prevalent in those over 40. Symptoms can include:

- Dry, burning or itchy eyes, nose and mouth (with increased dental decay)

- Vaginal dryness

- Sore or cracked tongue and dry or peeling lips

- Dry or burning feeling in throat

- Difficulty talking, chewing or swallowing

- Dry skin or rash

- Joint pain, stiffness or swelling

- Fatigue

Antiphospholipid Syndrome

In antiphospholipid syndrome, the immune system mistakenly attacks proteins in the blood, causing blood clots to form within arteries or veins of the kidneys or lungs or brain, which may cause deep vein thrombosis, a stroke, heart attack or pulmonary embolism, depending on the location of the clot. It is often the clinical explanation for repeated miscarriage. There is no cure, but medications can reduce the risk of blood clots.

Pregnancy-Related Risk Factors

Women who experience certain pregnancy-related complications are at an increased risk for heart disease. Some of these risk factors include:

- **Gestational diabetes**: Pregnant women who develop elevated blood sugar that first appears during pregnancy are said to have gestational diabetes. Generally, gestational diabetes resolves after delivery. However, women who have had gestational diabetes have a significantly higher risk of developing diabetes within five to 10 years after delivery.

- **Gestational hypertension**: This is high blood pressure that develops after week 20 of pregnancy but resolves after delivery.

- **Preeclampsia**: This is a serious condition of pregnancy characterized by high blood pressure and sometimes elevated protein in the urine. It usually develops after week 20 of pregnancy but can be diagnosed even after delivery. Preeclampsia can lead to serious complications if not treated in a timely manner. Women with diabetes and obesity before pregnancy are at an increased risk of developing preeclampsia. Although typically the symptoms go away after delivery, women who have experienced preeclampsia have an increased risk of developing high blood pressure later in life. Women who had preeclampsia during pregnancy double their risk for heart disease, and the more severe the preeclampsia, the greater the risk.

• **Eclampsia:** This is a rare and severe complication of preeclampsia in which there are seizures resulting in periods of disturbed brain activity that can cause episodes of staring, decreased alertness and violent shaking (convulsions). Eclampsia affects about one in every 200 women with preeclampsia.

Gestational diabetes, gestational hypertension, preeclampsia and eclampsia are all linked to an increased lifetime risk of heart disease, including coronary heart disease, heart attack and heart failure. It is important to tell your doctor if you had any of these conditions so your heart disease risk can be accurately assessed.

Know Your Score: Your Personal Risk Factor Assessment

All of the recent studies confirm that heart disease can be prevented or controlled with:

- Awareness, knowledge and ability to put into action those lifestyle changes that prevent or control the risk factors that lead to heart disease or that eliminate the issues that already caused a heart attack.

- Partnering with your doctor to develop a personalized plan for risk factor identification and modification.

- Adherence to all medically prescribed recommendations, including medications taken regularly, as prescribed.

The following questions will help you assess your personal risk of heart disease.

Your Personal Risk Factor Assessment

These are risk factors for heart disease you cannot control (*nonmodifiable risks*).

Circle Yes or No

1. Race and gender

I am Black or Latina or South Asian   Yes   No

2. Age

I am 55 years or older   Yes   No

3. Menstrual history

I am post-menopausal or had surgically   Yes   No
induced menopause

I went through menopause before the age of 40   Yes   No

4. Family history/genetics

I have/had a male relative who had heart disease   Yes   No
before age 55

I have/had a female relative who had heart   Yes   No
disease before age 65

These are risk factors you can control *(modifiable risks)*.

5. Pregnancy issues

During one or more pregnancies, I had   Yes   No
gestational diabetes (elevated blood sugar),
preeclampsia, eclampsia or elevated
blood pressure

6. Blood pressure

I am being treated for high blood pressure   Yes   No
or my BP was 140/90 or higher on two or
more occasions (or 135/85 if diabetic)

7. Diabetes

I have diabetes or I have been told my   Yes   No
blood sugar is high

8. Cholesterol

My cholesterol level is   _____

My HDL (high-density lipoprotein) is   Yes   No
less than 50 mg/dl

My LDL (low-density lipoprotein) is   Yes   No
greater than 100 mg/dl

My triglycerides are greater than 150 mg/dl   Yes   No

9. BMI

I have a BMI (body mass index) of 25 or more   Yes   No

10. Waist circumference

My waist measures more than 35 inches   Yes   No

11. Cigarette smoking

I smoke cigarettes   Yes   No

I live or work with people who smoke   Yes   No
cigarettes in my presence

12. Physical activity

I get less than 30 minutes of physical   Yes   No
activity on most days of the week

13. Autoimmune diseases

I have been diagnosed with rheumatoid   Yes   No
arthritis, lupus or other autoimmune condition

14. Stress/lifestyle

I feel stressed much of the time   Yes   No

I am always on the go with little or   Yes   No
no time for myself

I can get overwhelmed with a   Yes   No
sense of foreboding (doom and gloom)

15. Sleep

I routinely get less than seven   Yes   No
hours of sleep per night

Totals: Yes ____   No ____

Understanding Your Score

Look at your total score. Every *yes* in the category of modifiable risk factors indicates an area where you have an opportunity to make changes to get your health on track. We recommend that you take this list to your doctor along with your *Personal Health Inventory* so that he or she can help you customize a program that focuses on specific areas in which you need help. Your doctor can also fill in the blanks if you were unable to answer any of the questions, such as those asking for cholesterol or blood pressure numbers. Going forward, make sure you know these important numbers.

If you did mark *yes* to any of these questions, but are thinking, "I feel fine, why do I need to make any changes?" remember that heart disease begins silently and can remain hidden for years; you may not know the impact of your risk factors until it's too late. Our goal is to help make sure that does not happen to you. As we've mentioned throughout this book, it is never too late to begin your journey to heart health.

Risk Factors for Heart Disease in Women: a Recap

- Family history of premature heart disease in a first-degree relative, i.e., parent, sibling or child (before age 55 in a male relative, or age 65 in a female relative)

- Race or ethnicity (higher for Black, Latina and South Asian women)

- Age (higher for women over the age of 55)

- Prediabetes: HbA1c of greater than 5.7 percent

- Diabetes: HbA1c of greater than 6.5 percent

- Hypertension: higher than 120/80 mm Hg

- Abnormal cholesterol/triglyceride levels

- Obesity, especially where the bulk of weight is in the waist/ midsection ("apple shape")

- Cigarette smoking, or frequent exposure to secondhand smoke

- Physical inactivity (sedentary lifestyle)

- Early onset (before age 40) of menopause from any cause

- Stress

- Lack of adequate sleep

- Systemic autoimmune disease (e.g., lupus, rheumatoid arthritis)

- A history of pregnancy-induced diabetes, hypertension, preeclampsia or eclampsia

Now that you have the background, you are aware of the risk factors and have completed your personal assessment for heart disease, it's time to learn more about the clues and cues your own body is providing.

Pay Attention to the Clues and Cues: Your Body Tells a Story

Claudia

Remember Claudia, the 48-year-old woman we introduced in Chapter 1? As you will recall, Claudia is a high-level banker with a stressful career and a busy home life. As luck would have it, her symptoms of exhaustion, heart palpitations, shortness of breath and changes in her usually calm demeanor coincided with her annual checkup with her primary care physician.

Claudia described her diminished energy and other symptoms to her doctor. She performed a thorough examination, which included a complete battery of blood tests. Her doctor noted that this was the second time that her blood pressure had been elevated in the office and performed a treadmill exercise stress test to see if elevated blood pressure with exercise was the cause of her symptoms. After eight minutes on the treadmill the test was stopped due to Claudia's fatigue and very elevated blood pressure. Her doctor placed her on medications to control her blood pressure and recommended that she come back in three months for a follow-up visit.

Claudia resumed her busy schedule, took her blood pressure medication and gradually returned to exercising on the treadmill for 30 minutes a day, five times a week. She continued to have diminished energy, and she noted a slight change in her usually sound sleep pattern. Now she had trouble falling asleep and on a few occasions awakened suddenly, feeling anxious for no apparent reason. She attributed her sleep disturbance to anxiety about her upcoming trip to Hong Kong, where she was going to close a huge financial deal.

It was two months after her stress test that we met Claudia in the emergency room. On that day she had returned from her four-day trip to Hong Kong and had gone directly from the airport to her office. However, right away she began to experience overwhelming fatigue and severe shortness of breath. In addition, she was sweaty and had mild chest discomfort. She told her coworkers she was sure it was just jet lag, but they didn't agree and called 911.

Tests in the emergency room indicated an abnormal electrocardiogram (EKG), a sign that she might be on the verge of having a heart attack. A coronary angiogram (x-ray of the coronary arteries) revealed plaque in the heart's large coronary arteries, with a clot creating a significant blockage in a branch of one of the main arteries. At age 48, Claudia underwent an emergency procedure to place a stent (a small, tube-shaped device) in the artery to keep it open and increase blood flow to her heart, thereby avoiding the possibility of an imminent heart attack. As she lay in the recovery room, Claudia recalled that both her mother and her older brother had had a stent implanted, for similar reasons.

It is possible that Claudia's stressful schedule, the 14-hour flight with little sleep and dehydration precipitated the clot formation and led to the symptoms that brought her to the emergency room. But going to the emergency room and having the stent procedure performed less than three hours from the onset of her first symptoms probably saved her life! That blocked vessel could very well have caused a heart attack.

The sequence of events leading up to her emergency stent procedure made Claudia reflect on the important clues her body was providing that she had either missed completely or passed off as unimportant. She now understood that her body was signaling that something was seriously wrong. She realized that her mother's and brother's history of heart disease, her own elevated blood pressure and the constant stress caused by family life and work all placed her at risk for heart disease. Once she began experiencing a noticeable decrease in her ability to exercise, a feeling of fatigue while walking and episodes of shortness of breath for no apparent reason, she should have recognized that those were all clues and cues that she had heart disease – clues and cues that she ignored.

Trust Your Intuition!

Heart disease warning signs can be subtle. Women often ignore what they think are minor aches and pains, but you need to know that if something doesn't feel quite right, it probably isn't. Trust your intuition – make a doctor's appointment and get yourself checked out. If you suffer from one or more of the symptoms listed later in this chapter, it could be an early warning sign of cardiac disease. Call your doctor right away. Do not hesitate, because your life could depend on it.

Work with Your Doctor to Establish a Personal Baseline

There are many early warning signs of heart disease that often go unnoticed, and the best way to determine the significance of these symptoms is to visit your doctor. If you are having symptoms, and these symptoms are due to heart disease, you can be treated, and if they are not, then your doctor can use the visit to establish a baseline to assess any future symptoms. If you are not having symptoms, your annual well-woman visit will provide your doctor with an opportunity to screen you for any evidence of heart disease or heart disease risks (see Week 4 of the Six S.T.E.P.S. in Six Weeks Program). Being aware of how your body feels and functions when it is in a healthy state allows you to recognize anything you experience that is out of the ordinary. When you are tuned in to your normal everyday aches, pains, sleeping patterns and activity thresholds and are aware of how you normally react to work and family stress, you and your doctor will be more aware of and better able to judge the seriousness of any symptoms you may be experiencing, and you will be in a much better position to know when to consult your health provider.

Developing an ongoing partnership with your health care provider and knowing your baseline are of critical importance for all women, but especially for those of you who already have any of the risk factors for heart disease. If this describes you, be especially vigilant about monitoring your health and reporting any and all changes, no matter now minor you think they are, to your health care provider.

The Signs and Symptoms of Ischemic Heart Disease or Heart Attack

Recognizing the signs and symptoms of ischemic heart disease or heart attack may be challenging when it comes to women. Even today, when we know so much more about women's heart attacks, many doctors tend to focus on the most common symptom (in both men and women): chest pain or discomfort. But this is problematic for women, since most of them do not exhibit this symptom and therefore a heart attack can go undiagnosed. That is why you need to advocate for yourself and help your doctor diagnose your heart attack. It could save your life. Remember, too, that you can experience *any* of the common symptoms listed below, days, weeks or months before a heart attack actually occurs. Some of these symptoms may seem so benign that you want to brush them off. Don't. Seemingly benign symptoms like shortness of breath, a passing pain in the chest, heartburn, nausea and vomiting and back or jaw pain may not seem like emergencies, but if they tend to recur, call your doctor and get checked out. Always err on the side of safety.

The Most Common Symptoms for Women

While many men and women experience chest pain or chest pressure that radiates to the left arm as the main sign of a heart attack or of ischemic heart disease, the following symptoms are far more common in women than in men and can lead to an underappreciation by both women and their clinicians of the likelihood of heart disease. As you look at this list, it's important to remember that every woman is different; some may experience only one of the following signs, some may experience more than one sign and 40 percent may experience no chest pain at all.

- **Uncomfortable pressure, fullness, squeezing sensation or pain *anywhere in the chest or back.*** These symptoms may last only a few minutes or longer; they may persist or occur sporadically. None of these symptoms is normal in a healthy woman.

- **Mild or intense pain that begins in the chest and spreads to the shoulders, neck, jaw or arms** (left or right side). This type of pain is more common in women and can come on suddenly (and can even wake you up), or it can come and go before getting more intense.

- **Unexplained dizziness, lightheadedness, fainting.** These symptoms may or may not be accompanied by palpitations.

- **Shortness of breath or difficulty breathing with or without discomfort in the chest.** This feeling can be experienced alone or may be combined with nausea or lightheadedness.

- **Clammy sweating.** This is the type of sweating that comes with feeling anxious or stressed out; it feels different from sweating when you are experiencing a hot flash, are in a warm place or are exercising. Breaking out in a nervous/cold sweat is a symptom very common in women who are having a heart attack.

- **Stomach pain, abdominal pressure or nausea** that may feel like common indigestion, the flu or a stomach ulcer but can also feel like a weight sitting on your stomach.

- **Back pain** that may mimic muscle pain related to overexertion.

- **A feeling of weakness or fatigue or the inability to perform even simple tasks or activities.** The onset of any of these symptoms may or may not be sudden and without any obvious cause. They are sometimes combined with vague feelings of lack of mental sharpness and that something is "just not right."

When to Call 911

If you are experiencing these symptoms and think they may represent a heart attack, call 911! Time is a crucial factor when dealing with a heart attack. The sooner you get help, the better your chances of a full recovery. Call 911 immediately if you experience any of the above symptoms – no matter how subtle – and say out loud to yourself or anyone around you, "I think I am having a heart attack." Trust your gut feeling. Never second-guess yourself. Do not wait for the pain or strange feeling to pass.

Under no circumstances should you attempt to drive yourself or allow anyone else to drive you to the hospital. You need to be in an ambulance! The sooner you get medical help, the better your chances of survival. If you are having a heart attack, your treatment will start the moment the ambulance arrives. Your life may depend on it.

Then, before the ambulance arrives, if you know you can safely take aspirin, *chew* one full-strength aspirin tablet (or three low-dose tablets), with or without water. Sit down and rest until the ambulance arrives.

Honestly Evaluate Your Lifestyle to Make Meaningful Changes

Be honest with yourself. As you read earlier, Claudia believed that she was living a heart-smart life. She was careful to maintain an exercise regimen that included aerobic activity and strength training. She kept an eye on the scale to make sure her weight stayed within five pounds of her pre-pregnancy weight. She took good care of her appearance, and everyone told her how great she looked. Heart disease was not on her radar!

But what Claudia failed to realize was that she needed to be more honest with herself and to delve more deeply into her family history and her daily routine to see what she needed to change. Fortunately for Claudia, before she left the hospital the medical team helped her in this process. They helped her recognize that despite her exercising and her focus on weight, she had developed certain habits that contributed to her visit to the emergency room.

These habits included eating fatty "comfort" foods, such as steak, cheese, cookies and chips, when traveling. The constant stress of dealing with the competing demands of her job and family – long hours of travel, soccer games, homework and housework – had taken its toll. As if this wasn't enough, Claudia put pressure on herself to always bring her "A" game and to be as close to perfection as possible in everything she tackled. All of these things were major contributors to her heart disease.

With the help of her medical team, Claudia was able to develop a plan like the one you are about to learn that focuses on the important changes needed to prevent a heart attack.

When it comes to our approach to food, exercise, sleep hygiene and stress management, we can all make small changes in our daily routines and habits, and these small changes can yield meaningful results. As you will see when you read on, the Six S.T.E.P.S. in Six Weeks Program we have designed will jump-start your journey to heart-smart living. Like Claudia, you'll be surprised at how simple it can be. Let's get started!

Part Two

Six S.T.E.P.S. in Six Weeks to Heart-Healthy Living

"I have been impressed with the urgency of doing. Knowing is not enough; we must apply. Being willing is not enough; we must do."

—Leonardo da Vinci

Introduction to the Heart Smart Program

The goals of our Six S.T.E.P.S. in Six Weeks Program are to give you the tools to better understand your personal health status and to encourage you to partner with your physician and take an active role in your own health and well-being. We want you to feel empowered to make the small changes that can lessen your chances of ever developing heart disease.

It is important that your health is always your top priority, so we have designed a program that is easy to follow and easy to live with to help you accomplish that goal. Below is a synopsis of the program, which includes the area of focus for each week. The last week, Week 6, shows you how to put it all together and take permanent S.T.E.P.S. to your healthier life.

WEEK 1   **S**: Select and stock the kitchen with healthy food choices.

WEEK 2   **T**: Take control of your activity and choose to move every day.

WEEK 3   **E**: Eat for heart-healthy living.

- Set a healthy table.

- Eat healthy at home and when dining out.

WEEK 4   **P**: Partner with your doctor, family and friends.

WEEK 5   **S**: Sleep more, stress less and savor life.

WEEK 6   **Put it all together:** Permanent S.T.E.P.S. to Heart-Healthy Living

Before you start the Six S.T.E.P.S. in Six Weeks Program…

Choose a Buddy

The program is easy to follow, but because all journeys are easier and more enjoyable with the company of a friend or family member, we strongly encourage you to ask someone close to you to help on this journey. This should be someone who can offer you moral support and encouragement, share in your successes and provide a friendly ear if you are finding it difficult to stay on course; someone who can laugh with you and compliment you when you make progress; someone who can be counted on to share and celebrate your triumphs and prop you up when you slip. In short, someone who will always be there for you.

If you and your buddy are both working toward these same heart-health goals, you can share suggestions and solutions. Two people going through the same experiences together can have a very powerful and positive effect on each other.

Keep a Notebook/Journal/
Smartphone Log

A journal is the optimal tool to track your progress as you begin this health journey, and it will be helpful for years to come. Purchase a journal that you like and find easy to use, because it's going to be your lifelong companion. Treat yourself to a beautiful hard-cover journal or, just as good, pick up an inexpensive spiral notebook at the dollar store. Look for one with dividers to help you get organized. You can also set up your journal on your smartphone, computer or tablet. What matters most is the ease of use, to help you track your progress consistently.

This simple journal will become the most important asset on your road to a healthy heart in ways you can't yet imagine. Charting your progress will help you stay motivated. You'll find it a real eye-opener when you read back over your journal and see how far you've come. Keeping a record allows you to remember this entire journey – and document your accomplishments and challenges.

Part 1 of your journal includes your *Personal Health Inventory*, discussed earlier. It may take a little time to fill this section in now but it will be invaluable for years to come:

- Family medical history, including a general look at your family's health (e.g., mother had cancer at age 57, brother has had hypertension since age 43, etc.)

- Your medical history (pregnancies, surgeries, procedures and hospitalizations as well as chronic conditions)

- Allergies (including details about the type of reaction you may have had)

- Current medications and vitamins/supplements (including dosage and frequency)

- Previous regimens of medication, vitamins/supplements and all other over-the-counter products (including any reactions or side effects)

- Date of birth and, if relevant, age at time of menopause

- Race and ethnicity

- Smoking history

- Exercise habits (how many years exercising? how often?)

- Stress in your life

- Autoimmune diseases

- Pregnancy-related risk factors (gestational diabetes, gestational hypertension, preeclampsia, eclampsia)

- Recent medical tests (including HbA1c, blood pressure, cholesterol levels)

- Weight

- BMI

It's a good idea to set aside a section of your journal for listing the questions you want to ask your health care professional during your office visit or on the phone. Be sure to leave enough space to note the answers and any special instructions. It's not uncommon to forget our questions when we get to the doctor's office!

Bring your journal to all doctor's appointments. Even if you are seeing several doctors within the same health care system, your medical records might not be shared between physicians. You are responsible for keeping your medical team up to date, and the most efficient and effective way to do this is to provide them with the information from your *Personal Health Inventory.*

We suggest that you organize your journal so there is a section for each week of the program. Ideally, you should write in your journal every day of every week. This important tool will become a permanent record that will support your healthy life to come.

Try to keep your notebook updated. Note your progress, identify setbacks or successes and keep track of all questions or concerns you need to raise with your health care professionals. Be sure to set time aside to read over what you've written so you stay on track with your health and don't forget anything. You may choose to share your journal with your buddy for his/her input.

Before you start the program, as you should before starting any type of health program, *get checked out by a doctor or nurse practitioner*. Explain that you are starting a new program. When you go for this first visit, take your journal along. Be sure you've filled in your list of personal risk factors and as much of your *Personal Health Inventory* as possible. Armed with this information, you will be well on your way to becoming an active partner with your doctor.

Now, let's get started!

S: Select and Stock the Kitchen with Healthy Food Choices

To create a heart-healthy environment at home, and to be able to set a healthy table, you'll need to make decisions about choosing healthy foods. What you have in your house right now may not live up to heart-smart standards, so we will go through your kitchen, see what needs to be eliminated and then offer suggestions on what you can buy to replace those less healthy items.

Clean Out Your Refrigerator

The key to heart-healthy living is knowing which foods are good for you to eat and which are not. Take stock of the contents of your refrigerator. Do you find whole milk, butter, ketchup, salad dressings, fruit juice, sodas, high-fat leftovers (casseroles, pizza and desserts), lard, bacon, processed meats, fruit nectars, jellies and jams or marshmallow fluff? Check the freezer as well. There you may find more high-fat leftovers along with ice cream, ice pops, frozen pizza, fish sticks and more.

The foods that we just listed are the foods you are going to get rid of, because all are high in fat or sugar or both. Check the labels. Learn which foods in your refrigerator and freezer are "ultra-processed" foods and should be purged. Ultra-processed foods are foods that contain ingredients that are not typically used when cooking from scratch, such as artificial sweeteners, colors or flavors or other additives. Some examples of ultra-processed foods are soft drinks, many cereals, chicken or fish nuggets and instant soups, just to name a few. These foods are loaded with chemical additives and are often high in sugars, saturated fats and sodium, all of which contribute to heart disease. The bottom line is that these foods are generally high in calories and low in nutrients and have no place in a heart-healthy kitchen.

In most cases, there are healthier alternatives to all of these foods that will keep you satisfied and that you will enjoy so much that you won't miss the unhealthy foods you used to eat. But right now your goal is to get rid of all the harmful foods listed above. Any food that is high in refined carbohydrates, unhealthy fats or sugar should be purged from your kitchen. From now on, the goal is to focus on buying and eating flavorful, healthy foods.

Purge the Pantry

Now move on to the cupboards. Just as you did in the refrigerator and freezer, take a good look at what you've accumulated over the years (yes, years). Chances are, if you're like the rest of us, you will find packages of food that are older than your children! The best way to do this purge is to get a large trash bag and toss out the food with the expired dates. Take a separate bag and fill it with all of the unexpired foods you never got around to making or eating, and foods no one in the family likes or will eat.

More importantly, also rid your kitchen of the foods that are not expired and that you might like to eat but that don't fit into your new eating program. These foods, along with the unexpired foods mentioned above, can be donated to a local food bank or community center. This includes things like: pretzels, chips of any kind (potato, taco, corn, veggie, etc.), packaged cookies, cakes, pies, cake or cookie mixes, full-fat baking mixes, etc. You get the idea. All of the ultra-processed foods in your pantry should be purged. Packages of baked goods, snacks and desserts are generally ultra-processed, but check the label's first three ingredients. If some form of added sugar or fat is listed in the top three, it no longer belongs in your house.

Create Your Healthy Food Makeover

Now that you have purged your refrigerator, freezer and pantry of the unhealthy foods, it's time to restock your home with healthy foods.

Foods that belong in your new and improved kitchen include:

- Plenty of fresh fruits and vegetables

- Whole-grain breads, pasta, crackers, flour, cereals

- High-fiber foods like beans, dried peas, lentils and chick-peas ("pulse" foods)

- Brown rice and other whole grains

- Raw, unsalted almonds, cashews, pecans and walnuts

- Unsalted sunflower and pumpkin seeds

- Low-fat or fat-free dairy products

- All-natural peanut and nut butters

- Eggs and/or packaged egg whites or egg substitutes

These foods are healthier versions of the foods that you already eat.

Your Heart-Smart Shopping List

Below is a detailed list of suggestions, but more and more healthy options appear on the grocery shelves every day, so read those labels. You'll be surprised at the available variety of food that is good for you. It might take a few tries to find the brands you and your family prefer, and they may cost a bit more, but it's worth the investment. Once you discover healthy new foods that you enjoy, you will never feel deprived. Please do not give up! We have found that this new way of eating sometimes take a little getting used to. It might be just that you are unaccustomed to less sugar, salt and fat in your diet. So be patient while your taste buds adjust.

Dairy and Eggs

From now on, choose to eat low-fat or fat-free skim milk and dairy products or milk alternatives such as soy milk and milk made from nuts (almond, cashew, etc.) or rice, to name a few. If you are buying cow's milk, stay away from the "whole" or full-fat variety. That also goes for cheese and yogurt. Today's low-fat, skim and fat-free varieties of milk, cream, half and half, sour cream and yogurt and reduced-fat cheeses taste surprisingly good and are just as nutritious as their full-fat counterparts.

If you are lactose intolerant or just prefer one of the plant-based "milks," you are lucky to be living in a time where you can choose a milk made from soy, almond or rice, among others. Some of these taste like the milk we all know and some are flavored (avoid the ones with added sugar), which add a nice touch to cereal or a cup of coffee. Again, try different brands until you find the ones you like best.

While you're in the dairy section, don't forget eggs. The latest research says that if your LDL cholesterol is within healthy limits, you do not have to eliminate the yolks as long as you eat eggs in moderation. However, if you have trouble maintaining healthy LDL cholesterol levels, or if you have diabetes, then try to limit yolks to three per week. Also, remember to prepare your eggs without added saturated fats and avoid eating them with high-fat foods such as bacon or toast with butter.

We find that it's always good to have a container of egg substitutes on hand (and an extra container in the freezer), as they are versatile. You can scramble them or make an omelet, and you can use them in baking and cooking. The word *substitute*s is a bit of a misnomer, because these products are really egg whites that have been made to look like whole eggs.

Meat, Poultry and Fish

Meat, poultry and fish are high in protein and other important nutrients and are an integral part of a healthy eating plan, so leave room in your freezer to stock these items. The only concession you'll need to make is to limit portion size (see Week 3), but meat, poultry and fish can still be part of your life.

When it comes to meat, choose the leaner cuts, like top or bottom round, pork tenderloin or boneless pork chops and ground meat that is 85 percent or leaner. Stay away from the fatty meats, which include pork bacon, ribs, pork shoulder chops and roasts, marbled steaks and chuck roasts. Lamb is also a good option when you choose lean cuts from the leg and loin. Avoid cuts from the rib and shoulder blade, which are higher in fat. A three-ounce cooked lean cut of meat contains, on average, less than 10 grams of fat, less than 4.5 grams of saturated fat and less than 95 milligrams of cholesterol.

Fish should definitely be a part of your diet; we recommend eating it at least twice a week. All unprocessed fish is good, but focus on eating mostly "high-trophic" (fatty) fish like salmon, mackerel and herring because they are higher in omega-3 fatty acids, as opposed to low-trophic fish like catfish or crawfish. Canned fish is also a healthy choice, so stock up on mackerel, sardines, salmon and tuna. But a word of caution: Watch how you prepare the fish. For example, don't fry fish and turn a healthy dish into an unhealthy one. Other unhealthy forms of fish are fish sticks and prebreaded varieties, which are often high in added sodium and added fats. Steaming, grilling, baking and broiling are all preferred ways to prepare fish.

Most types of shellfish are a good choice for lean protein since they are low in saturated fat. Clams, oysters, mussels, scallops, lobster and crab are low in cholesterol. However, some varieties of shellfish are high in cholesterol. Shrimp contain the highest amount of cholesterol among the shellfish, about 166 mg per three ounces. However, new guidelines suggest that dietary cholesterol has little effect on blood cholesterol, so moderate consumption of any type of shellfish should not be a problem. The issue with shellfish is that it is often pre-pared with ingredients high in saturated fats (think shrimp or lobster in cream or butter sauce, or fried fish and chips). Avoid frying shellfish and cook it in a healthier way, with lit-tle added fat and without rich cream and butter sauces.

While fish is a heart-healthy food, there are some concerns that we want to address. Some species are overfished and some are high in heavy metals and toxins. While we encour-age you to consume fish regularly, it would be wise to select fish that are sustainably sourced and are not high in mer-cury and other toxins. Stay away from swordfish, shark, king mackerel, gulf tilefish, marlin and orange roughy, which are all high in mercury. Certain farmed fish, such as farmed salmon, contain polychlorinated biphenyls (PCBs), which may contribute to cancer risk. The following website is help-ful for determining if a fish is a good choice and sustainably sourced: www.seafoodwatch.org.

Poultry is another good choice, but when it comes to ground chicken or turkey make sure you buy the brand with the low-est fat content, and remove the skin on whole chicken parts before eating.

These days the many varieties of sausage made from either turkey or chicken rival the pork varieties for taste. Try them; we're sure you'll be pleasantly surprised. Don't forget, too, about turkey bacon.

Fruits and Vegetables

Fruits and vegetables are chock full of vitamins, minerals and fiber and have proved beneficial in preventing or treating disease. Fresh, frozen or canned (low sodium) are all great choices. When buying canned fruit, make sure it's packed in natural juices or water. Keep your refrigerator full of raw vegetables and fruit for healthy snacking and add fruit to every meal, breakfast, lunch and dinner. There are no bad choices when it comes to this food group. Remember, too, that some vegetables, like the leafy green varieties (kale, spinach, Swiss chard, broccoli rabe, etc.), are also high in iron and will taste great in a fruit salad.

Whole Grains, Beans and Lentils

Grains and beans are plants and can also be considered vegetables, but because they are so crucial to a healthy diet, they are highlighted here. Whole grains, beans and lentils should all be part of your diet. With a focus on eating healthy whole foods, check out the tasty grains that are also healthy carbs that add fiber. Quinoa, spelt, flax, chia, barley and farro are all ancient grains that are making a comeback as part of the thoroughly modern diet. When it comes to pasta, steer clear of high-carb varieties and try the newer whole-grain versions, which have gotten a lot tastier over the past few years. Look for pastas that are made from 100 percent whole grain. Remember to stick to recommended serving sizes, because pasta is a type of carb you can easily overeat.

When buying bread, cereal, pastas and flours, always choose high-fiber, whole-grain varieties. If you buy white flour, make sure it's unbleached. When it comes to rice, stay away from white and choose brown rice or another type that hasn't been stripped of its bran layer. If it has a color, it's the better choice. When choosing a nutritious, high-fiber cereal, you cannot beat that old standby, oatmeal, especially the steel-cut variety. If you buy the instant oatmeal, make sure it is the plain variety with no added sugar, which many instant varieties have. You can always add your own fruit, such as bananas, apples, peaches, pears or berries (fresh, dried or frozen) or raisins, and/or a sprinkle of cinnamon to make it tastier without adding sugar.

It goes without saying that fried chips (potato, taco, corn and their cousins) are not part of a healthy diet – even if they are whole grain. One reading of the label will tell you they are much too high in fat and salt.

Beans (including the canned variety) are an excellent component of a healthy diet. Beans are nutrient dense (meaning they have high amounts of nutrients per calorie), are high in protein, carbohydrates, vitamins and minerals and are low in fat. If you are eating canned beans, remember to rinse them well to remove as much salt as possible.

Condiments/Flavorings

Some condiments are high in sugar or fat. Ketchup, for example, can be very high in sugar, but there are now some low-sugar varieties available. The same goes for salad dressings and barbecue sauces, which can be high in both sugar and fat. Mayonnaise shouldn't be a worry unless you eat an excessive amount in dressings. You can also choose one of the healthier varieties made with canola or olive oil. For salad dressings, read the labels and choose the lighter varieties, or get used to using a smaller amount. Better yet, make your own. Fruit jellies and jams and preserves also fall into this category, and all traditionally made varieties are almost half sugar. For this reason we suggest buying the fruit-only varieties. They taste exactly the same. Excellent condiment choices are mustard, salsa and hot sauce, which tend to be fat free and can be used to dress up a variety of foods.

Salt

To add flavor to foods, don't rely on the salt – in fact, we suggest that you take the salt shaker off the table! We get enough sodium in our diet naturally from food and from those hidden sources of sodium in packaged or prepared foods. To bump up flavor, try a salt substitute, cook with garlic, use lemon juice and lemon zest and don't be afraid to experiment with spices and herbs. Try one of the many packaged spice and herb combinations (but make sure to read the label and only buy one with no added salt), or make your own.

To recap, the condiments we recommend stocking in your refrigerator or pantry are:

- Mustard

- Ketchup (low or no sugar)

- Vinegars (balsamic, apple cider, etc.)

- Salsa

- Hot sauce (including sriracha)

- Dried spices without additives (such as cinnamon, thyme, basil, parsley, red pepper, cumin)

- Tahini

- All-fruit jellies or jams

- Lemon zest

Beverages

When it comes to nonalcoholic beverages, the choices are pretty simple:

Anything containing sugar is out. This includes any full-sugar sodas, fruit nectars and fruit juices. You should be eating fruit, not drinking it. If you prefer to have a flavored beverage, that's not a problem. You'll find many fruit-flavored and no- or low-calorie sparkling waters on the supermarket shelves. Or make your own soft drink by splashing a bit of fruit juice into a glass of plain seltzer, squeezing in a wedge of lemon, lime or orange or infusing other fresh fruit or vegetables. Cucumber water is particularly refreshing!

Drinking diet soda is not a good idea. If you can't give up diet sodas and beverages completely, limit what you drink to one or two per week, because many recent studies actually link diet soda consumption to weight gain as well as high blood sugar.

Coffee and tea are back on the recommended food list, and caffeine isn't an issue unless it keeps you up at night. Flavored and herbal teas are always a good choice, as is green tea with its own health benefits.

To sum it up, the following beverages are your best choices, because they hydrate without added sugar or calories:

* Water (add flavor with a spritz of citrus, or infuse with fruit)

* Sparkling water or seltzer

* Unsweetened coffee or tea

When it comes to alcoholic beverages, red wine has recently been given the distinction of being a heart-healthy addition to the diet. Red wine contains polyphenols that may reduce the risk of stroke and heart disease by protecting the lining of the blood vessels in your heart. However, it is important to note that this means "moderate" wine consumption, which for women is one five-ounce serving per day. It is not recommended that you start drinking wine if you don't already do so, and if you do drink, don't increase the amount you drink. If you abstain from alcohol, you can get heart-healthy benefits from other sources of polyphenols, such as green tea, grapes or grape juice (limit to four ounces of juice), and even a small square of dark chocolate of 70 percent cacao content or higher.

With respect to other types of alcohol such as beer and hard liquor, avoid drinking to excess. Too much alcohol has been associated with raising triglycerides and contributing to weight gain and obesity. And most cocktails are prepared with a lot of sugar. If you choose to drink, avoid sugary cocktails and instead choose one serving of the following: wine (five ounces), beer (12 ounces) or hard liquor (one ounce).

Sweeteners

It is best to limit the amount of refined white sugar in your diet. However, sometimes we all need a little something sweet! *We recommend that you steer clear of all artificial sweeteners and sugar substitutes.* If you are cooking or baking, there are many all-natural sugar substitutes, some of which even provide nutritional benefits. Some recipes can be altered by replacing part of the sugar with molasses, agave, honey or maple syrup (real, not artificially flavored). These ingredients behave somewhat differently from sugar, so you may have to do some research or use trial and error to find the right balance.

Oils, Butter and Buttery Spreads

Monosaturated oils such as olive, canola, peanut and safflower are all heart healthy. A fruity olive oil can be pricey, but it is healthy and deliciously tasty in a salad dressing, or when used sparingly as a substitute for butter. Make sure to select extra-virgin olive oil that has been cold pressed to get the most polyphenols and superior taste. For cooking without added fat, use nonstick sprays.

We've never met a person who didn't like butter, but butter consumption should be limited. A little dab is okay here and there, but don't overdo it. A pat of butter has 2.2 grams of saturated fat, and you should aim to use less than 15 grams total of saturated fat per day. You may think margarine is a better choice, but stick margarines contain partially hydrogenated oils, and some tub margarines have just as much saturated fat as butter. Although margarine does not contain cholesterol, it does contain fat and calories. If you opt to use margarine, read the label and choose the one with the lowest saturated fat.

Heart-Smart Pantry Staples

Below is a list of staples that we recommend adding to your shopping list to help you stock your new heart-healthy pantry. This list is by no means complete, but it will guide you in choosing the healthy foods to have on hand so that you can create a range of well-balanced meals or treat yourself to a healthy snack.

- Flour, unbleached

- Whole-wheat flour

- Cornmeal

- Cereals (oatmeal and any other cereals with five or more grams of fiber, three grams or less of fat and eight grams or less of sugar per serving)

- Whole-grain bread/crackers

- Brown rice

- Whole-grain pasta

- Whole-grain side dishes (quinoa, spelt, flax, millet, farro, barley, etc.)

- Spaghetti sauce (low sodium, low or no sugar)

- Canned tomatoes (whole, diced or pureed)

- Honey, agave, maple syrup, molasses

- Coffee and tea

- Soups and broths (low sodium)

- Canned fish (salmon, herring, tuna, sardines and mackerel) packed in water, olive oil or tomato sauce

- Oils for cooking and salad dressings (olive, canola, safflower)

- Beans and lentils (dried and canned)

- Fruits and vegetables (fresh, canned or frozen)

- Ketchup (low sugar)

- Mayonnaise (olive oil or canola oil)

- Mustard/salsa/hot sauce (to dress up meat, fish, potatoes, eggs)

- Salad dressings (low sugar/light)

- Vinegar (for homemade dressings)

- Pickles

- Fruit spreads (low or no sugar)

- Healthy snacks (whole-grain pretzels, crackers, graham crackers)

- Almonds, cashews, pecans, walnuts (raw, unsalted and plain dry roasted)

- Nut butters with no added sugar or salt (almond, peanut, cashew or sunflower)

Grocery Shopping Tips

Shop the walls: Produce, meats, fish, dairy, bread and deli products are stocked along the outside walls of the supermarket. When you shop the perimeter of the store you won't be tempted by the unhealthy foods that you are trying to avoid. If you must pass through the bakery department, pick up some tasty whole-grain bread as you are breezing through.

Always read the labels: Many packaged foods have surprising amounts of sodium, sugar and/or fat. For example, spaghetti sauce, bread, cereal, yogurt and marinades can have added sugar. If you see any of the following listed on a food label, know that the body processes all of these as sugar, because that is what they are: maltose, fructose, high-fructose corn syrup, dextrose, lactose, sucrose, molasses, cane sugar, corn sweetener, raw sugar, white granulated sugar, brown sugar, sugar, powdered sugar, invert sugar, fruit juice concentrate, applesauce, syrup, honey, malt syrup, maple syrup, nectars!

Make a shopping list: Make a list, buy only what's on it and don't browse! Doing this will save you money, calories and time. It's also a good idea to list your purchases in categories and in the order in which the foods are arranged in your particular market. Use your computer to make up a blank template that you can print out and fill in with what you need before you go to the store. Or go to your local supermarket chain's website; you may find one ready to use that can be filled out by clicking on the selected items.

Eat before you go shopping: Have you noticed that it's difficult to stick to your shopping list if you're hungry? Try to do your food shopping *after* you eat your breakfast, lunch or dinner. Don't "stop for a couple of items" on your way home from work if you are hungry. Go home and eat dinner and then go back out to the store – you'll save money and calories.

Stock up: If you can, shop for the coming month. The idea here is to develop your own system of planning meals and then shopping for the ingredients. When you stock up, you'll always have groceries on hand and will be less likely to run out for fast food. Now that you've cleaned out the pantry and know what foods you need to eat, get the family involved and plan ahead.

Demonstrate healthy eating habits: Getting healthy is a family affair, and you are all going to be eating the same food. (Granted, the kids may still get an occasional sugary snack, but limit these to teach them healthy eating habits.)

Get family members involved: Chances are your family members have a favorite type of food that they cook well, so you can enhance the cooking and shopping experience by assigning a day of the week to cook for the family to each member of your household who wants to cook. Your role will be to point out some healthy options. For those who are too young to cook, ask for their suggestions and get them involved by shopping and maybe even helping with the preparation – even if it's only setting the table. These types of activities that are centered around meals encourage family members to become active participants in creating, cooking and serving heart-healthy foods they like to eat, and you get the bonus of having the family sit down together for a meal.

If you live alone, buddy up with a couple of friends or relatives and cook for each other. In this case, the choice of meal is up to the cook. Or, each of you can make a meal and package and freeze it for each member of your group. Set aside a day to exchange these preportioned meals so that each of you will have multiple heart-healthy meals in your freezer.

Create a meal-planner notebook: We have found that using a loose-leaf notebook or a program on your computer that has dividers or tabs you can designate for breakfast, lunch, dinner, desserts and snacks will help you keep track of your favorite recipes as well as the ingredients needed to prepare them. Doing this offers the added advantage of providing space to write comments on the recipe, such as "Mary really liked this" or "Easy to make."

Now on to Week 2, and let's talk about that other essential element of your lifestyle that will keep your heart healthy: adding exercise to your daily routine.

T: Take Control of Your Activity and Choose to Move Every Day

Now that you have stocked your pantry with heart-healthy foods, it is time to incorporate a daily activity routine into your heart-healthy lifestyle. In this chapter, we will focus on three types of activity:

- **Walking:** The health benefits of aerobic activity and how to meet your goals

- **Strength and Flexibility Training:** The importance of strong and flexible muscles

- **Moving:** The significant health benefits of choosing to just "move" more in your everyday activities

Even if you don't plan to join a gym or devise a formal exercise program to follow at home, you do need to ensure that aerobic activity, strength and flexibility training and simply moving more throughout the day are all part of your life.

Research has shown that the simple act of walking is "the closest thing we have to a wonder drug," according to Dr. Thomas Frieden, former director for the Centers for Disease Control and Prevention. In order to maximize the health benefits of walking, incorporate a good walk into your daily routine. We encourage you to add other types of aerobic activity to your daily life. Pull out that old bicycle (the one you rode around the neighborhood when you were a teenager, or the stationary one that now sits idle in your bedroom closet) and go for a spin. The same goes for that treadmill gathering dust. Consider joining a gym or going to an exercise class. The purpose of this chapter is to give you a framework and some suggestions to get you on the road to incorporating these three elements into your daily life: walking, flexibility and strength training and just plain moving.

Focusing on your heart health means embracing a more active lifestyle and in the process discovering the incredible benefits of activity. The great thing about being more active is that you will experience the benefits almost immediately. When you are active, your body is moving in a higher gear, your heart is beating faster and oxygen-rich blood is being pumped through your body and nourishing your organs and your brain. You think more clearly, sleep better and have more energy. The more energy you expend, the more you will have. Your joints will lubricate and your muscles will stretch – and you'll feel better physically, emotionally and mentally. Being more active will energize your life.

But first things first! As mentioned, be sure you get a checkup from your doctor before you begin any type of exercise program – including a walking regimen. Your doctor or nurse practitioner will let you know if you have any limitations, and if you do, pay attention to them and don't try to push past them. As you build stamina your threshold will increase. Be patient.

Walking

The Benefits of Walking

All of us learn to walk as toddlers, so by now you have decades of experience with this "wonder drug." We agree that it is the perfect way to get your daily dose of activity.

Numerous studies confirm the health benefits of walking. One important example is the landmark Harvard Nurses' Health Study, in which the health behaviors of over 200,000 women were studied for more than 30 years. This study showed that walking at a moderate pace for an average of 30 minutes each day can lower the risk of heart disease, stroke and diabetes by 30 to 40 percent, and the risk of breast cancer by 20 to 30 percent.

If those statistics don't convince you to lace up your walking shoes and head out the door, here are a few additional facts about walking:

It helps to lower blood pressure, improves balance and bone strength (thereby reducing the likelihood of falls and fractures), counteracts the effects of weight-promoting genes, improves sleep, boosts your mood and sharpens your thinking. Best of all, walking is gentle on your knees – and the rest of your body.

Consider this: An eight-year study of more than 70,000 women found that brisk walking and vigorous exercise substantially reduced the incidence of heart attacks. What's more, even light to moderate activity – a minimum of one hour a week – was associated with lower rates of heart disease. We can all do that. But increase that number to 30 minutes per day and your risk of premature death will be significantly lower than if you didn't exercise at all.

Setting Goals for Your Walking Program

Your goal should be to work up to walking 30 minutes each day at a pace that is "moderate" or "purposeful." Think of the pace at which you would walk to a meeting if you were running a few minutes late; a pace at which you could carry on a conversation, but with a bit of difficulty. In that way, you will get your heart rate up and will experience the benefits of aerobic activity.

What is aerobic activity? Aerobic activity is sometimes referred to as "cardio," and it includes any brisk activity that stimulates and strengthens the heart and lungs, thereby improving the body's use of oxygen.

How to Begin a Walking Program

The Physical Activity Guidelines from the U.S. Department of Health and Human Services recommend adults get 150 minutes of moderate aerobic exercise each week, and we want you to target that amount as your ultimate goal. However, for those of you who have not been exercising on a regular basis, we recommend starting slowly – and checking with your doctor before you do. Begin with three to five minutes of moderate or "purposeful" walking each day. This should translate into three to three and a half miles per hour in order to get your heart rate to where it should be. Be sure to warm up and cool down for two to three minutes.

After you have completed week one of your walking program, increase the purposeful walking component by five minutes, and continue to do that each week until you reach 20 minutes of purposeful walking each day (with an additional five-minute warm-up and a five-minute cool-down). For those of you who prefer to count how many steps you are taking, we recommend starting with 3,000 steps and gradually working your way up to 10,000 steps each day.

Listed below are some easy ways to get in your 30 minutes of walking every day:

- Take a walk after dinner or lunch.

- Take public transportation one stop before or beyond your usual stop.

- Walk before work or walk to work, if that's possible (ditto the walk home).

- Enlist a family member or neighbor to join you for a walk.

- Walk your dog or volunteer to walk a neighbor's dog.

- Take the long route when walking anywhere (including the mall).

- Join the morning walking group at your local mall (call the mall to get the time).

- Head to the local elementary or high school and walk around the track.

It's important to remember that significant benefits are to be had even if you are not able to meet these goals. Any additional activity is a *step* in the right direction! Just to recap, the benefits of walking each day are:

- Lowered blood pressure

- Reduced risk of heart disease and certain types of cancer

- Increased joint and muscle strength and flexibility

- Increased bone strength

- Increased energy level

- Improved sleep

What to Wear: Dress for Comfort and Safety

Dress for the temperature, but be sure you have good socks and shoes and a bra that supports you well. Everything you wear has to fit well, be comfortable and not bind or chafe. Walmart, Kmart, Target and thrift stores all sell good work-out clothes. Just don't skimp when it comes to walking shoes. Good shoes keep you in balance by supporting your ankles, knees and back, and they also make your feet feel good, and that's important. You need the benefits of a walking program to maximize your health, so buy the best pair of shoes you can afford!

Safety Tips

We can't repeat these often enough:

When walking during hot weather, dress in lightweight and light-colored clothing.

Don't forget to wear sunscreen and sunglasses.

Never leave home without a cell phone.

If walking after dark, wear reflective clothing and/or a clip-on light and/or carry a flashlight.

Make sure you always tell someone where and when you will be walking and when you expect to be back. So many people forget this step!

Enlist the company of a friend or family member to make walking more enjoyable and safer.

Adhere to the rules of the road by using sidewalks and crosswalks and obeying traffic signals.

When on rural or suburban roads, always walk facing oncoming traffic (unless you are walking up a hill or around a blind bend) so you can see what is coming and have time to get out of the way, if necessary.

Always walk in familiar places where you know you will be safe.

Learn to Monitor Your Heart Rate

As we mentioned earlier, it is important to get approval from your doctor or nurse practitioner before beginning any exercise routine. Once you have the go-ahead, you will need to learn how to monitor your heart rate to ensure that you are getting the most out of your workout. If you are new to exercise, you may not be accustomed to the feeling of your heart working at increased capacity. You may feel that you are getting lots of exercise as you go up and down stairs at work or walk around the mall, but unless you properly monitor your heart rate, you won't know for sure. Depending on a number of physical factors including weight, overall health, muscle condition and blood pressure, you could be working your heart too hard, or not hard enough, without even knowing it.

Know How Hard Your Heart Is Working

You can't tell how hard your heart is working by how much you sweat. Even while working out at the same intensity, some women are drenched while others are barely damp. Heart monitoring calculates the intensity of your workout by actually counting the number of heartbeats per minute (BPM). Exercise makes the heart beat faster, making it work harder to deliver the increased blood and oxygen demanded by the muscles during a workout.

To exercise safely you should stay in a "zone" between 50 and 85 percent of your *maximum target heart rate,* which is defined as the absolute highest rate a heart should beat during exercise at a specific age. As a general rule, your maximum heart rate is approximately 220 minus your age.

Unless you are a professional athlete in training, your heart should never beat as fast as the maximum rate. Because heart rate is related to age and because the heart slows slightly as we age, our target zone beats per minute will decrease as we age. Below is a chart* to help you determine your target heart rate zone, counting beats per minute:

Age	Target Heart Rate Zone	Maximum Heart Rate
20	100-170 BPM	200 BPM
30	95-162 BPM	190 BPM
35	93-157 BPM	185 BPM
40	90-153 BPM	180 BPM
45	88-149 BPM	175 BPM
50	85-145 BPM	170 BPM
55	83-140 BPM	165 BPM
60	80-136 BPM	160 BPM
65	78-132 BPM	155 BPM
70	75-128 BPM	150 BPM

*Reference: American Heart Association www.heart.org/HEARTORG/HealthyLiving/PhysicalActivity/
FitnessBasics/Target-Heart-Rates_UCM_434341_Article.jsp#.WZ8iqz6GPmF

Knowing your range helps you determine how hard you should be exercising and when you are overdoing it – or not pushing yourself enough. When first starting your exercise regimen, aim for the low end of the zone, and as you build stamina and add more intense workouts, aim for the higher end of the zone.

How to Measure BPM

Every beat of your pulse is a beat of your heart. The easiest way to accurately count the number of times your heart is beating per minute is to check your pulse. Gently place your forefinger and middle finger on the inside of your opposite wrist. Hold your finger there for 15 seconds, counting the beats. Then take that number, multiply it by four and you will have your BPM.

You should take your pulse periodically as you exercise.

Strength and Flexibility Training

As we now know, aerobic activity is essential for good heart health. However, in order to ensure that you embark on an exercise program designed to improve your overall health, it is important to add some resistance, or strength, training as well as flexibility exercises to your weekly routine. This will help you build muscle mass, strengthen your bones and improve your metabolism. Strength training enhances the benefits of aerobic exercise. It is important to include 20 to 30 minutes of strength and flexibility training in your exercise routine at least two times per week.

To begin your strength and flexibility program, you will need a few basics:

Equipment

Exercise/yoga mat: A soft surface will make exercising more comfortable. You can purchase a mat at a discount or sporting goods store.

Weights: Many strength-training exercises can be done with no equipment at all! Using only your own body weight, you can do planks, push-ups, wall push-ups, squats, abdominal crunches and more. But if you would also like to use weights for strength training, we recommend two dumbbells (two to five pounds each). If you don't have dumbbells, then take two empty one-liter soda bottles and fill them with water or sand. Better yet, use two plastic half-gallon milk bottles (with convenient handles, which make them easier to hold on to and manipulate). To make them lighter, reduce the amount of water or sand; you can add it back as you gain strength.

If you do decide you want to use dumbbells, by all means get them. You needn't purchase new ones. They can often be found in a thrift or used sporting equipment store. Initially, five pounds each should be your limit. They may not seem heavy enough, but once you start lifting them multiple times, you will see that they are!

Resistance bands: These are stretchable bands that provide resistance when stretched. You can find them in any sporting goods store.

For suggestions on a simple strength-training workout that can be done almost anywhere, with no equipment other than a chair and your body weight, see Appendix B, Strength and Flexibility Exercises.

Flexibility Exercises

Stretching is an important part of any exercise routine. It is recommended that you perform flexibility exercises for all of your major muscle groups: upper body (shoulders, chest, arms) and lower body (glutes, adductors, hamstrings, quadriceps and calves). In Appendix B we have provided some suggestions for flexibility exercises for each of these major muscle groups.

Moving – 10 Minutes at a Time

Even if you are a seasoned exercise buff, if you look for them you can probably find more opportunities to move throughout the day. The goal is to take every opportunity to keep your body *moving*, rather than remaining sitting or standing still. Prolonged sitting can be damaging to your health even if you already exercise on a regular basis. Here are some suggestions, which we hope will get you thinking of even more ways to add movement to your day:

- Park your car farther away from your office, the bank, the store, etc.

- Pace the room while you're on the phone or watching TV.

- Stand up and march in place each time a commercial comes on.

- Take the stairs instead of the elevator or get off a floor or two earlier (or more, if you are able) and walk the rest of the way.

- Walk up the escalator or along the moving sidewalk – don't stand still.

- Use the bathroom one floor up or down at work and take the stairs.

- Get up from your desk at least once every hour to stretch your legs for a minute or more.

- Do a few minutes of yard work (pull a few weeds, rake a bit, sweep the walk).

Remember to Hydrate

Making sure you drink enough water is always important, but remember to drink even more when you exercise. The body can become dehydrated for a number of reasons. Sweating is the major reason during exercise, but you can also get dehydrated when it's cold outside and you are not sweating. Exercise causes the body to dehydrate no matter what the temperature.

So make it a point to drink an eight-ounce glass of water about 10 minutes before you walk or exercise and another glass or two when you finish, no matter what the season or temperature. In addition, you should get into the habit of always having a bottle of water handy to sip throughout the day, no matter what the temperature and no matter where you are, to help you stay hydrated.

Set Aside a Specific Time and Place to Exercise

Choose any time of the day that works best for you and when you won't feel pressed for time. For indoor exercising, find a place where you have the space to lift your weights and keep your "exercise stuff" together. The point is to make this as easy and fuss free as possible. You need to be able to just walk to your space and start exercising. Maybe there is space in front of your TV – if so, consider doing your workout while watching your favorite show. Do whatever it takes to make this as enjoyable as you can.

There are many videos and books to help you map out a personalized exercise routine. We recommend Mayo Clinic Fitness for Everybody, which contains 150 easy-to-follow illustrated exercises and is available online through www.amazon.com or www.bookstore.mayoclinic.com.

Log Your Progress

Keeping track of your exercise progress will prove invaluable to you on your road to heart health. Not only will you be able to look back and see how far you've come, but it will also make it easier to set realistic goals for yourself as you continue with your exercise program. Record keeping will encourage you to keep going and to take pride in your accomplishments. There are many different ways to log your progress, so choose the one that works best for you. For example:

In Your Journal

Use your trusty journal. Add a section to keep track of your strength-training progress, and simply note the number of reps you do for each exercise, gradually increasing the number of reps (until you reach 10 to 12) or the amount of weight (if you are using dumbbells or ankle/wrist weights).

If you are walking, it might help to use a pedometer or download an app on your phone that counts your steps.

Remember that you are counting all of your steps during the day, not only the time you actually go out for a walk. Up and down those stairs, back and forth to the kitchen and bathroom, to and from your car – all those steps add up. Aim for 3,000 steps a day to start and increase gradually until you get to 10,000 (about five miles) per day. (Figure that there are roughly between 2,200 and 2,300 steps per mile.)

You can also download a walking journal or workout template from the internet. Search for "free walking log," "free walking journal" or "exercise log" and you'll be directed to many sites where you can choose the type of log or journal format you prefer, print out the blank template and insert it into your journal. If you aren't computer savvy, ask your children or friends to help you. You may inspire them to keep a log, too.

Electronically

Keeping track of your walking progress is effortless if you wear an activity tracker, pedometer or smart watch or use a phone app that electronically maintains a log for you. All that is required is an initial setup of the application or device. If you want to buy an activity tracker but aren't exactly sure if one is right for you, read on and also check them out in person at any sporting goods, electronics or department store.

The biggest boon to fitness in general and walking in particular is the tracker. Perhaps you've seen these brightly colored rubber bracelets with flashing lights on people's wrists. A basic tracker (which generally sells for between $50 and $100) is preset to a goal of 10,000 steps, or five miles per day. But that number can be adjusted higher or lower, depending on where you are in your walking goals. They can be a great motivator and may be worth the investment. In addition to counting steps, these basic trackers can monitor hours slept and keep track of calories and ounces of water consumed. More sophisticated models alert for email or text messages, tell time, monitor heart rate and count number of stairs climbed or laps swum. The Apple Watch, at the more expensive end, is almost as smart as a smartphone. But a basic pedometer works perfectly well if your goal is just to count steps.

When you opt to wear an exercise tracker, you will have an easy way to keep an accurate record not only of how many steps you've taken but also of the duration and intensity of your movement. This way you will know just how much of your walking is moderate or purposeful as opposed to simply strolling.

These devices take the guesswork out of keeping track of your movement, but they cannot do the work for you. What they can do, however, is motivate you into action and keep you going. What the trackers and apps can do and the pedometers cannot is – via your computer, smartphone or tablet – maintain a log of your daily activity, monitor your progress and reward you when you've met your goals. In addition, some new ones even reward you with "prizes" when goals are met or exceeded.

Like to be social? Some trackers and phone apps allow you to incorporate social networking elements so that you and your friends, colleagues or family members can register on their website as a "group" that will post progress of each member. If you aren't comfortable with having people you know see your progress, you can be measured against strangers who have registered but wish to remain anonymous as well. This friendly competition can prove to be a real motivator.

If you already own a smartphone and don't want to go to the expense or keep track of another electronic device in your life, then download one of the many free apps. Many have monitoring capabilities similar to those of the fitness trackers, and some are more sophisticated than others. Don't be afraid to try out different ones until you find the one that best suits your needs.

If you're turned off by the appearance of the solid-colored rubbery wristband, there is good news! Check out the Internet and you will find beautifully colored and decorated wristbands for many varieties of trackers, most modestly priced at just a couple of dollars. Some are more sophisticated in their design and actually look like bracelets, which makes them wearable with even the trendiest outfits. Who knew?

Once you get hooked on the positive feedback you get from your device, it will be hard to stop wearing it. Twenty-four hours a day, this little device is capable of motivating you and keeping track of how much you've slept, how much ground you've covered, how many calories you've eaten and burned, how many pounds you've lost, how far away you are from your target weight, and they even reward you when you reach daily or long-term goals. If you have had trouble motivating yourself to exercise, a fitness tracker may provide the push you need to get going. If you're the competitive type, it will keep upping the ante and raising your goals. No matter how you look at it, these devices make striving toward a healthier and more active life easier.

But the bottom line is that whatever device you opt for – or whether you opt for a journal instead – you still need to put in the miles yourself. So, start moving!

Other Types of Exercises

Although our focus here is on walking, strength training and flexibility exercises, there are countless other activities that can provide an excellent workout. Jogging, swimming, cycling, rowing, tennis, skating, skiing and basketball are just a few aerobic activities that will contribute to your heart health. Learn to monitor your pulse while you engage in these activities to ensure that you are within your target heart rate zone.

Summary

The most important advice for you to take away from this section is that **any movement or activity that you add to your daily routine is beneficial to your heart health.** If you have not previously included exercise as part of your daily regimen, slowly work up to the goal of 30 minutes of moderate aerobic activity each day, with additional twice-a-week strength and flexibility exercises. Start slowly, and gradually build on your progress from the day before. Keep track of your progress and note what works for you and what doesn't. Most importantly, enjoy yourself…and, better yet, be proud of yourself!

Now, on to Week 3, and eating heart smart.

E: Eat for Heart-Healthy Living

Because the subject of eating is of such major importance when it comes to maintaining heart health, Week 3 is presented in two parts. We have separated the basic guidelines for setting a healthy table from the rules for healthy eating, both at home and dining out.

Part 1 – Set a Healthy Table

At Week 3, your kitchen is in good shape and exercise is becoming part of your daily life. So, let's now turn to the subject we all love – eating. In the first section, we focus on the basic rules for healthy eating and how to do that without denying yourself your favorite or comfort foods. You will see how easy it is to eat in moderation and prepare familiar or traditional foods in healthy ways. You'll also learn which foods are best for keeping your heart healthy and your body satisfied.

Healthy Eating:
Eating to Live, Not Living to Eat

We all need to eat in order to stay alive, but when we live to eat – well, that's what gets us in trouble. However, eating to live also means knowing how to choose tasty foods that will be calorie friendly and good for our blood pressure, arteries and any health conditions we may have, such as diabetes, heart issues or obesity.

This sounds simple, but if you already have health problems, you probably have a complicated relationship with food that interferes with making healthy choices. Our health depends on the foods we choose to put in our bodies. What we eat can either harm our health or keep us healthy. All the medicine in the world can't overcome the effects of an unhealthy diet. But once you know the basics for making healthy food choices, you'll be on the road to heart health.

Why Eating Is Emotionally Complicated

Many of us come from families that equate food with success and happiness. We all had a mother, grandmother or aunt who wasn't happy unless we ate everything on our plate, whether we were hungry or not. Perhaps they told you stories of the starving children who would have gobbled up the food left on your plate. Or maybe you learned to "medicate" with food – when you were unhappy, perhaps an ice cream cone, a slice of cake or pie or a candy bar made you feel better. If you felt lonely, maybe eating a dish of spaghetti, macaroni and cheese or a pepperoni pizza did the trick. We all have our traditional favorites, and we tend to eat them in large portions and not always cooked in a healthy way. Complicated relationships with food are common, and it is often not until we get older that we begin to understand the health consequences attached to not paying more attention to what we put in our mouths.

Our goal is not to analyze all of the psychological forces at work when it comes to your eating habits. But we can help you prepare, serve and eat familiar and satisfying foods in healthier ways and in healthier portion sizes, which will improve and maintain your heart health.

Your New Adventure

You've heard these rules before: eat whole foods, eat a plant-based diet, do not eat ultra-processed foods, do not eat fried foods, eliminate added sugar and reduce our intake of fat. However, putting these rules into practice takes some getting used to. Cooking by these new rules means that some of your favorite foods may not taste the same, but trust us – you'll get used to the new tastes, portion sizes and ways of cooking. Once you start noticing a difference in the way you feel and look, you'll never go back to the old ways.

Eating Healthy at Every Meal: Six Basic Steps

1. Skip the Second Helpings!

It doesn't matter how healthy your diet is; if you eat too much you will gain weight. So from now on your two watchwords are *moderation* and *balance*.

It's easier to overeat these days, because portion sizes have gotten larger over the years. For example, in the 1970s, soda was sold in eight-ounce bottles. As time went on, the portion size increased to 12 ounces and then was "supersized" to 20 ounces, an increase of over 145 calories! In 1990, an average bagel was three inches in diameter (approximately 145 calories). Today's average bagel is five to six inches in diameter (approximately 350 calories), more than double the original in calories. The problem is that these big portions now seem normal!

When you eat at home, put a moderate-size portion of food on your plate at the kitchen counter or stove, and don't return for seconds. When dining out, eat only what you know to be a sensible portion and then ask for a doggie bag. You'll have a meal for another day.

From this point on you need to pay attention to the size of your meals and also to the space taken up on your plate by each type of food. That way, you won't need a scale or calorie counter for the task. (See Appendix G for some easy and fun ways to "eyeball" healthy portions of various foods.) You'll develop this skill fairly quickly, and it will help you to portion out your meals at home and eat less when dining out.

2. Eat a Wide Variety of Plant-Based and Whole Foods

Fruits, vegetables, grains and legumes tend to be low in fat *and* cholesterol in addition to being excellent sources of fiber, complex carbohydrates, vitamins and minerals. Nuts and seeds are also nutritious plant-based foods that are high in fiber, vitamins, minerals, protein and healthy fats. Don't forget, however, that the amount of nutrition you get from these plant-based foods depends on how they are cooked. Frying any vegetable, for example, turns a healthy food into an unhealthy one.

When preparing your dinner, make sure most of your plate is devoted to plant-based foods. Remember that brown rice is better than white, whole grains are better than refined, lightly steamed veggies are better than mushy ones and green salads are always a healthy choice (as long as you go easy on the dressing, or leave it off completely).

Fruits and vegetables are also high in fiber – also known as roughage – which is good for your digestive tract, and eating them can help lower cholesterol. Fiber is the part of the plant that cannot be digested, but it absorbs many times its weight in water, resulting in softer, bulkier stools. A high-fiber diet keeps food moving through the system and keeps you feeling fuller with much less food. Fibrous food also takes longer to chew and slows down the pace of eating. The slower you eat, the less you eat, because it takes time for the brain to get the message from the stomach that it is full. Although it's always important to drink enough water, it's doubly important when eating foods high in fiber to prevent constipation.

There are two types of fiber.

Soluble fiber. This type of fiber is partially broken down in water and can actually help lower cholesterol. Oatmeal, oat bran, barley, nuts, seeds, legumes (such as all dried beans and lentils) and fruits contain soluble fiber. So pass up the orange, grapefruit, tomato and other juices and eat the whole vegetable or fruit instead.

Insoluble fiber. This type of fiber cannot be broken down in water and does not lower cholesterol, but it is still important to your diet as it promotes normal bowel function. Whole grains, such as those found in whole-wheat bread, brown rice and bulgur, or any grain that hasn't had its bran and germ removed by milling, all contain insoluble fiber and are also a great source of nutrients.

Many vegetables also contain insoluble fiber. Fresh or frozen carrots, zucchini, celery, tomatoes, broccoli, pumpkin, squash, cucumbers, cabbage, Brussels sprouts, turnips and cauliflower are good choices. Try to stay away from canned vegetables, especially if you have high blood pressure, because of the amount of salt they contain. If this isn't possible, buy the low-salt brand or rinse well before heating.

Maximize the amount of insoluble fiber in your diet by selecting packaged grains, such as bread and English muffins that are made from whole grains (whole wheat, whole oats, etc.). If the label doesn't specifically list whole grain as a main ingredient do not buy it.

3. Institute Meatless Mondays and Eat Fish Two Times a Week

The "meatless Mondays" movement is an easy way to help cut down on eating high-fat protein (like red meat) and boost your intake of plant-based foods that are rich in antioxidants and fiber. Simply eliminate meat from your meals one day each week. This will help you expand your cooking repertoire so that you may eventually be able to cook more adventurous and tasty no-meat meals. But, in the meantime, start out by trying to do without meat one day each week.

If you're not one who enjoys vegetarian dining, eating fish is a great way to get the benefits of protein without adding fat and cholesterol to your diet. Fish is also high in omega-3 polyunsaturated fatty acids, which greatly reduce the risk of developing coronary artery disease. Omega-3s help decrease cardiac arrhythmia, lower triglyceride levels, slow the buildup of plaque in arteries and slightly lower blood pressure. All fish contain this healthy fat, but salmon, mackerel, sardines, trout, bluefish, albacore tuna and herring are especially rich in omega-3s. The American Heart Association recommends eating at least two three-ounce servings of these types of fish each week in order to reap the health benefits.

Again, as with vegetables, frying destroys the health benefits of fish, as does adding creamy sauces. Grill, bake, broil or poach fish. Add a little olive oil and season with lemon and garlic (before or after cooking) for a simple, delicious and healthy meal.

4. Eat at Home More Often and Cut Back on Eating Processed Foods

Nothing is getting more press these days than the health risks of eating processed foods. Although it was possible to eat only unprocessed foods – like meat, fish, poultry, eggs, fruits and vegetables – in times gone by, it's impossible to completely eliminate processed foods from the modern diet. Below are some suggestions for eating as healthy as today's lifestyle will allow. Stick to these guidelines and an occasional meal at a fast-food venue won't be a major health risk – although even fast-food restaurants offer many more healthy choices today.

- Eat home-cooked meals as often as you can. This way you will control how your food tastes and what goes into making it.

- Limit the size of your portions.

- Put your fork down between bites to encourage yourself to eat more slowly.

- Cut down on eating heavily processed foods. Many pantry staples – bread, pasta, cereal, soups – are processed. Cook what you can from scratch and buy the healthiest versions of those you are unable to cook yourself.

- Make eating enjoyable. Share meals with friends and family. If you have children living at home, try to get everyone together for a meal as often as you can – and leave the cell phones in another room! Human interaction is also good for your health.

- Don't forget to drink! Drinking any type of nonalcoholic beverage, especially water, seltzer and other nonsweetened beverages, is important to keep the organs running smoothly and to prevent dehydration!

- Eat a variety of foods. Variety really is the spice of life, so change it up! It also sets a good example for the young ones in your life to be exposed to different foods and tastes.

- Eat slowly, and stop when you are full. It's okay to leave food on your plate.

- Eat well-balanced meals. They are healthy and satisfying.

- Choose healthy snacks. When you need a snack, choose a piece of fruit over that donut you hear calling your name!

5. Cut the Salt, Sugar and Saturated Fat

Salt is a major cause of high blood pressure and other related heart diseases. We now know that cutting salt in the diet reduces the risk of heart attacks and stroke. This is yet another reason to eliminate processed foods, because one of their major ingredients is what is referred to as hidden salt. Over 80 percent of salt intake is from processed foods. The American Heart Association encourages shoppers to become salt detectives by reading labels and only eating foods with 140 milligrams or less of sodium per serving, and we agree!

Tips for cutting salt:

- Eat only canned, frozen or other types of processed foods labeled "reduced sodium," "sodium-free," "no salt added" or "unsalted."

- Eat only foods with total sodium content of 140 mg or less per serving, if you can't get salt-free. Note that sodium may also be listed as MSG (monosodium glutamate).

- Eat steamed, grilled, baked, boiled and broiled foods and keep sauces, dressings and cheese "on the side." Be sure to make this request when ordering out.

- Eat high-sodium condiments sparingly. These include soy, steak and Worcestershire sauces, flavored seasoning salts, pickles, olives, anchovies, sauerkraut and salted tomato and vegetable juices.

- Season food with pepper, garlic, lemon or herbs and spices instead of salt. Salt-free seasonings are fine, but some seasoning blends do contain salt, MSG or salt products, so read the label.

- Check the hot sauce label. The original red tabasco sauce is low in sodium, but many hot sauces are not.

- Rinse canned meats, vegetables, beans and capers well in plain water to remove some of the sodium.

- Limit or eliminate consumption of cured meats, bacon, hot dogs, sausage, bologna, ham, salami, salted nuts and cheeses.

- Use margarine in moderation, because even though it contains less saturated fat than butter and no cholesterol, one tablespoon still averages about 150 mg of sodium.

Sugar is purely empty calories with no nutritional value. Eating food and drinking beverages containing large amounts of sugar are directly related to an increased risk of Type 2 diabetes, which in turn increases the risk of stroke and coronary artery disease. All sugary drinks and foods are high in calories and tend to be low in vitamins and minerals, so they fill you up quickly but will not leave you satisfied. This will tempt you into eating more than you need.

We do need some sugar in our diet, and sugar does occur naturally in food. For instance, fruit has fructose and milk has lactose, both natural sugars. The problem comes when we (or the food manufacturers) *add* sugar. These days, most of the sugar we eat comes from processed foods, which is another reason not to eat them. Also be aware that fat-free salad dressings, barbecue sauces, flavored yogurt, jarred spaghetti sauce, granola bars, ketchup and sweetened cereals all contain sugar. Be aware, too, that honey and fruit juices are still sugar, and the body reacts to them the same way it does to any sugar.

The American Heart Association recommends that women limit added sugars to no more than 100 calories per day, which translates into about six teaspoons (24 grams).

Tips for cutting sugar:

- Don't buy or eat foods that have any type of sugars listed as one of the first four ingredients. Note that sugar is listed in many ways: sucrose, glucose, fructose, maltose, dextrose, corn syrup, high-fructose corn syrup, brown sugar, raw sugar, molasses, concentrated fruit juice and honey.

- Eliminate all sugared drinks. Sugary carbonated drinks are the single largest source of calories in the American diet. One 12-ounce can of cola contains more than nine teaspoons (39 grams) of sugar! Attempting to quench your thirst with sugary beverages also means you will then drink less milk and other healthier beverages (like water or unsweetened green tea).

- Eat whole fruits and vegetables instead of drinking them. Fruit and vegetable juices and nectars are high in sugar (and sometimes sodium) and low in fiber and are much less satisfying.

- Eat candy in moderation. If you crave candy, choose dark chocolate and eat a piece or two to satisfy your craving, but stop there. Dark chocolate with 70 percent cacao content or higher has been shown to have some health benefits, but only if eaten in moderation. Make that candy bar last a few days!

Over the years, *fats* have developed a reputation that is unfair and unwarranted; the truth is that some fats are actually essential to a healthy diet. In fact, 25 to 35 percent of your daily calories should come from healthy fats. These fats are found in nut butters, vegetable oils, fatty fish, nuts, seeds, avocados and olives. They help the body absorb certain vitamins and help with appetite control, because eating fats can keep you from feeling hungry and overeating. Good fats are also helpful in preventing heart disease and certain cancers and relieving arthritis pain.

However, there are some fats you should avoid eating:

Saturated fat. This fat is a dietary demon because it raises LDL (bad) cholesterol, a major factor in heart disease and stroke. The American Heart Association recommends that saturated fats make up no more than five to six percent of an adult diet. As we said earlier, you do need to eat some fats to live, but they should be in the form of monounsaturated or polyunsaturated fats.

Tips for cutting saturated fat:

- Eat only lean cuts of beef, lamb, pork and poultry without skin and trim as much visible fat as you can from all types of meat before cooking.

- Consume only low-fat (1 percent) or nonfat milk and dairy products.

- Skim the fat off meat-based soups, cooling them in the refrigerator to solidify the fat so that it is easier to remove.

- Substitute canola, grapeseed or olive oil or nonstick spray when cooking and sautéing instead of using butter, lard or bacon grease.

- Steam vegetables or cook them in low-salt broth or diced tomatoes, instead of sautéing or deep frying.

- Switch to eating soups made from protein-rich legumes, such as kidney beans, black beans, pinto beans, lentils, split peas and chickpeas, instead of meat.

- Dress your salads with vinegar (or lemon) and oil or use only a tiny amount of a bottled brand to minimize consumption of fat, sugar and sodium.

- Eat plain steamed vegetables or eat them raw dipped in a little low-calorie salad dressing or salsa. You will be surprised how good they taste.

Trans fats. These are the truly bad fats, because they raise LDL (bad) cholesterol and lower HDL (good) cholesterol by making blood platelets stickier. Sticky platelets accelerate the progression of atherosclerosis and increase the risk of heart attack and stroke. Trans fats were unleashed on us by food companies who invented them to make sure their processed snacks, chips, cookies, baked goods and other foods stayed fresh as long as possible. They did this by taking essentially healthy monounsaturated and polyunsaturated fats and altering them by a process called partial hydrogenation, which makes them solid at room temperature. Because there is no safe limit for trans fats, eat them as infrequently as possible. This should be easy, since they are found mostly in snack foods! Although butter is not a trans fat, we still recommend limiting your butter consumption.

One last thing about trans fats: Labels can be misleading! Foods with less than 0.5 grams of trans fat per serving can *legally* claim to be trans fat free. This means that if you eat more than one serving of a food mislabeled in this way, you will actually be eating a significant amount of trans fats. If the label says "partially hydrogenated oil," don't buy it *or* eat it.

Tips for cutting trans fats:

- Replace the solid fats in your diet – margarine, lard and shortening – with liquid canola, grapeseed or olive oil or nonstick spray.

- Top your baked potato with salsa or low- or nonfat sour cream, yogurt or cottage cheese – not butter or margarine.

- Spread your whole-grain toast or muffins with all-fruit spreads or one of the buttery spreads described below – not butter or margarine.

- Bake your own low-fat, low-sugar cakes, cookies and pastries.

- Limit eating any baked goods and foods made with partially hydrogenated or saturated fats, including pies, donuts, crackers and French fries.

A special note about margarine, oil, butter and buttery spreads:

Margarine. Made from vegetable oils and containing no cholesterol, margarine is also higher in "good" fats – polyunsaturated and monounsaturated – than butter. But not all margarines are created equal, and some are even unhealthier than butter. This is especially true with hydrogenated margarines (which most are) because they add trans fats. So when you choose a margarine a good rule to remember is that the "harder" or more solid the margarine the more trans fats it contains. So always choose tub varieties over solid sticks.

Liquid vegetable oils. Throw away the lard and bacon fat and use only healthy oils like canola, corn, safflower, soybean and olive oil for cooking. These add no more than two grams of saturated fat per tablespoon.

Butter. Butter is made from milk, which comes from animals, and that means that, like meat, it can clog arteries and affect heart health. You should limit butter in your diet, but that doesn't mean you have to miss the taste. There are healthy substitutes.

Buttery spreads. There are now a variety of plant-based spreads in the dairy case alongside the butter and margarine. These products contain phytosterols, a natural plant compound that may reduce LDL (bad) cholesterol when eaten in recommended amounts and as part of a heart-healthy diet. The spreads taste good and can also be used in cooking and baking.

6. Eat Colorful Foods

The American Heart Association recommends that you "color your plate" to prevent heart disease. Your heart-healthy dinner plate will not only taste good, it will be satisfying and pretty to look at. Here's how to do it:

- Fill your plate with foods from all the major groups with an emphasis on colorful vegetables, fruits and whole grains.

- Experiment with different foods and cook up a storm with the wonderful assortment of fresh and frozen vegetables and fruits now available year round.

A registered dietitian or your doctor can help you determine how many portions of fruit and vegetables are right for you, but here are some daily guidelines: As part of a total 1,800-calorie diet, eat two cups of fruit, two and one half cups of vegetables and six whole-grain products (such as pasta, rice, quinoa, cereal, whole-wheat couscous or a slice of whole-grain bread) per day.

7. Replace the Foods You Love with Healthier Versions

In this day and age there is no reason to deprive yourself of the tastes you love in order to eat a healthy diet. What you've eaten in the past may have caused health problems, but there is no reason you cannot enjoy the same tastes in healthier versions. Even though some of these substitutions may not taste exactly the same at first, trust us, they really aren't that different and they do taste good. They'll be better for your family, too. In this chapter we've already suggested healthier alternatives for some foods, but on the next page are some additional suggestions.

Instead of...	Try...
Full-fat soft and whole-milk cheeses (e.g., colby, cheddar, brie, Velveeta, pimiento and most packaged or presliced varieties)	Nonfat, 1 percent or soy varieties (small amounts of full-fat cheese on an occasional basis are fine)
Fat- and sugar-filled dairy products (milk, ice cream, yogurt, cottage cheese, cream cheese)	Nonfat, low-fat or soy products
Cream of Wheat or farina	Regular or steel-cut oatmeal (not instant)
Mayonnaise	Light or low-sugar varieties
Premade salad dressing	Reduced-calorie dressings, fat-free dressings or homemade dressing with oil and vinegar or lemon juice and herbs
White potatoes	Yams or sweet potatoes
Eggs	Egg whites or egg substitutes
White rice	Brown or whole-grain rice

Instead of...	Try...
Sugary cereals	Bran or other whole-grain, low-sugar cereal
White sugar	Natural sugar substitutes in moderation A reduced amount of sugar for baking and cooking, substituting with fruit
Soda (including diet), fruit juice, nectars	Plain, sparkling or flavored water, or unsweetened iced tea
Pasta	Whole-wheat or veggie-based pasta
Salted nuts	Raw almonds, cashews, pecans or walnuts
Beef and pork	Fish, skinless chicken, tofu, beans or very lean cuts of beef or pork
Butter	Soft buttery spread (no trans fats) Olive oil (great on whole-grain toast)

Part 2 – Healthy Eating at Home and Dining Out

Now let's put your food knowledge into practice. Some rules will differ when you are dining out because you may need to think on your feet and make substitutions for what is available on the menu. In this regard, restaurant eating presents more of a challenge than cooking for yourself. Some of what you read in this chapter will reinforce what you learned in earlier chapters, as some rules bear repeating. Are you ready?

Presenting Your New Plate!

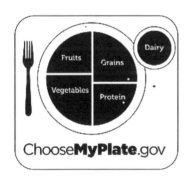

Whether you are eating at home or in a restaurant, this is what your plate should look like. This simple graphic was designed by the U.S.D.A. to remind Americans how easy it is to eat healthfully. So from now on, this is all you need to know to balance your food choices and avoid overly large portions.

- **Half the plate** is filled with fruits and vegetables. The proportion of each is up to you. Just make sure your selections take up half the plate.

- **One quarter of the plate** is filled with lean protein – lean meat, skinless chicken, fish or tofu.

- **One quarter of the plate** contains sweet potatoes, brown rice or whole grains.

- **The eight-ounce cup** or glass contains water, low-fat milk, sparkling or flavored water, unsweetened iced tea or other non-sugary, no-calorie beverage.

Serving Sizes

Dinner plates can vary in size, making it difficult to determine an appropriate portion size. For more specific information on how much of each food is considered a healthy serving, we have provided a guide in Appendix G.

Healthy Cooking Suggestions

Now that you know the types and quantities of foods that you are going to eat, here are some suggestions for cooking that food in ways that won't add sugar, salt, fat and calories.

- Add flavor with garlic, lemon juice, herbs and spices as a substitute for salt.

- Don't forget the pepper. Black pepper, hot pepper (sauce, fresh or ground), smoked paprika and chilies all add flavor and, depending on the pepper, a new dimension of heat.

- Limit meals with meat and poultry, and eat fish at least twice a week and vegetarian at least once a week (Meatless Mondays). Try turning your favorite meat dishes into vegetarian versions, such as vegetable lasagna, chili or pasta sauce.

- Use a rack when roasting poultry or meat so it doesn't sit in its own drippings.

- Don't baste meat or poultry with drippings. Instead use wine, low-salt stock, tomato or lemon juice.

- Grill or roast vegetables to bring out their natural sugars. Be careful not to overcook. Cut them to a uniform size, toss with one tablespoon of olive oil per cup of vegetables and roast on a cookie sheet or on the grill until tender.

- Use olive and canola oil for cooking, dressings and marinades.

- Add unsalted nuts (almonds, walnuts, hazelnuts, pecans, cashews, pistachios) to your daily diet by eating a handful or sprinkling them chopped or whole over salads, pasta and vegetables.

- Creatively add vegetables to meals and snacks. Add chopped vegetables to omelets and fruit smoothies, eat salads for lunch and dinner and pile sandwiches with cucumber slices, leafy greens, pepper rings, onion slices and tomatoes.

Plan Ahead

Cooking and eating most of your meals at home (and packing a healthy lunch for work) require planning ahead. You will need to be organized and keep an up-to-date shopping list posted where those in your household can write down what they want or what needs to be replaced. In addition, these suggestions can help you get dinner on the table with a minimum of fuss:

- *Cook your favorite foods.* Cook what you like. If you are dealing with an old family favorite, chances are it needs to be updated. Those old recipes tend to be high in salt, sugar and fat, so update them for your new, healthy lifestyle. Get creative.

- *Buy a new cookbook.* There are lots of great cookbooks that focus on health. Get one and add a few new dishes to your menu – it'll be like trying out a new restaurant.

- *Cook ahead.* Either set aside time at the beginning of the week or use any time you can find to cook more than one meal. That way, all you have to do is heat and serve. Many dishes (like chili, stews and soups) are much better tasting if not eaten immediately after they are made.

- *Prep your meals.* For meals that can't be made ahead, at least peel and cut up the vegetables, skin and/or bone the poultry, marinate meat or fish or precook what you can. Having part of the meal prepared means more time in the evening to relax.

- *Make double and freeze one.* This works especially well when making a pasta sauce, soup or casserole. Or, make your own "TV dinners" and keep a supply in the freezer. Thaw frozen meals in the fridge for 12 to 24 hours before you cook or reheat them.

- *Precut vegetables (and fruit) for snacks:* Carrots, celery, cucumbers, steamed broccoli, asparagus and apples are all good. Use hummus or salsa as a dip.

How Not to Overeat at Home

Overeating can be an issue if you live alone (or eat alone). Once in a while, invite friends over to join you, or gather the family or your significant other at the dinner table. But even with people around it's easy to sneak in that extra mouthful or to snack while cleaning up. So beware of these pitfalls when eating at home:

- *Limit alcohol.* Limit alcohol to one five-ounce or less glass of red wine *per day*.

- *Don't "sample" while cooking.* A small taste to adjust seasonings is fine, but excessive tasting or snacking while cooking can seriously increase the number of calories you consume.

- *Don't "pick" while cleaning up*. Same reason as above!

- *Eat only what is on your plate and do not go back for seconds.* Keep the serving dishes off the table. Better yet, serve the food directly from the cooking pots. Pack up what is left in the pots for another meal.

- *Use smaller plates.* It may surprise you, but this really works! Today's plates are much larger than the ones we used growing up. If you don't have any of those old plates in the back of the cupboard, ask your mother, aunts or siblings. If that doesn't work, buy a couple at a thrift store or use a "salad" plate as your dinner plate.

- *Eat slowly.* This is why it's good to have company. Talking makes the meal go more slowly. It takes time for your brain to catch up with your stomach. You can be full, but your brain won't know it if you eat too fast.

- *Stop when you are full.* If you aren't able to finish your meal, don't force yourself. However, if you find you have no appetite for a few days in a row, call your doctor.

- *Don't watch TV or talk on the phone while eating.* Pay attention to your meal. If you are distracted you won't be totally aware of how much you are eating (another reason to plate the meal in the kitchen).

Snacking

From time to time everyone needs a snack. Below are some suggestions to help get you through those times when your cravings take center stage.

- Use sliced cucumbers, tomatoes or zucchini as "chips." Top with low-fat cheese or cottage cheese.

- Eat a small sweet potato sprinkled with cinnamon. This will be a satisfying mid-afternoon or evening snack.

- Premeasure all snacks. Since snacking is usually done in front of the TV or while otherwise distracted, don't sit with an open package of any snack food (even if it is a healthy one), because you will lose track of how much you have eaten. Break down packages of snack foods into individually portioned bags. It's also more cost-effective to do it yourself than to buy them premeasured.

Dining Out

The same rules apply to dining in a restaurant or eating at someone else's house. Once you are not responsible for the preparation of your meal, ingredients and portion size may not be consistent with your new, healthier lifestyle. Here's how to make any meal healthier, even if you don't cook or serve it yourself:

The Three Major Temptations of Dining Out		
One	**Two**	**Three**
You have an entire menu – appetizers, entrees and desserts – with no limit as to what you can order. And a bottomless breadbasket!	Additional calories, salt, fat and sugar are added to many dishes in the form of sauces, gravies, toppings and condiments.	Portion sizes are generally significantly larger than what your body needs.

Tips for Overcoming the Three Major Temptations

First: If possible, review the menu online before you go to the restaurant. That way, you will not be making choices on the spur of the moment. If that is not possible, take a good look at the menu before you make your selection and don't be afraid to ask the server questions, such as how the dish is prepared (since it's not always obvious from the menu). Make substitution requests if needed. As a first step, eliminate the unhealthy foods such as anything pan- or deep-fried, scalloped (cooked in cream sauce), au gratin (cooked in cheese sauce) or stuffed (you never know every ingredient in stuffing, and the server probably doesn't know, either).

Second: It's the norm for salt to be added to restaurant food, so ask that no salt be added to your food. Concentrate on anything that is steamed, broiled, baked, grilled, poached or roasted. But you still need to ask the server if any of these foods are cooked in butter, have butter added or are served with a sauce, gravy or topping. If so, it doesn't mean you shouldn't order it, but it does mean that you should request that these calorie-laden extras be served "on the side." That way, you can use them sparingly and still enjoy the flavor they provide. Most restaurants are happy to oblige. Or, to add more flavor to your dish, ask for extra lemon, especially for fish or seafood.

Third: If you don't see a selection that fits the bill for you, ask them to make you one that does. Requesting broiled fish or chicken is not unreasonable, nor is asking that vegetables be steamed and served without butter, or that the potato be baked instead of mashed or fried. Most restaurants will comply with reasonable requests. Besides, we bet you aren't the only diner making them!

Additional Restaurant Recommendations

The Buffet! Nothing – we mean nothing – is as dangerous as the restaurant buffet table. The trick to healthy buffet eating is to fill up by eating the healthy foods first, which will leave less room for the dangerous, full-fat, empty-calorie desserts. With buffets you'll need to exert some extra effort to adhere to your healthy eating plan.

- Sail past the bread to the salads and fill your plate to the brim with healthy lettuce and vegetables, nuts and fruit. Top your salad off with minimal dressing or plain vinegar or lemon.

- Try a cup of the tasty soups available, especially the clear or vegetable-based ones, not the creamy ones.

- Choose protein wisely by staying away from all meats, poultry and fish that are floating in sauce or gravy and opt for those that look as close as possible to what you would prepare for yourself at home.

- Opt for the plain rice, the baked or boiled potatoes or a tiny plate of pasta. Remember, only a quarter of your plate should be devoted to carbs.

- Select vegetables that aren't swimming in butter. If that isn't possible, have another helping of salad.

- If you must splurge on dessert, eat one, but don't go back for seconds, unless it's fresh fruit, which should have been your first choice! Granted, you may have trouble getting past the dessert table, but there's no law against sharing one, or eating only half.

Remember the salad option and choose salads wisely. Adding a piece of broiled chicken to a specialty salad is always a good go-to option. This makes for a satisfying meal that fills out your plate perfectly, and it allows you to eat a piece of that delicious restaurant bread. However, read the ingredients carefully; many restaurants add dried fruit, bacon, marinated vegetables, pasta and other cured meats to their meal-size salads. Even smaller dinner salads can arrive dressed up with bacon bits – an ingredient you're better off not eating. Always ask what is in the salad so you are not surprised. Only use the house dressing if it is prepared with olive oil and be sure to ask for the dressing on the side so you can control how much of it you eat – or dress your salad with vinegar or lemon juice.

Tiptoe through the appetizer minefield. Appetizers are especially dangerous! Since you are usually hungry when you get to the restaurant, many appetizers sound delicious. It's the same principle as going food shopping when you're hungry. Looking over a menu of appetizers on an empty stomach is never a good idea – you will want them all! One way around this is to eat a small snack before you leave for the restaurant, such as a piece of fruit or some raw vegetables. You want to take the edge off your appetite. To keep your restaurant meal on track, try starting your meal with a simple salad or a vegetable-based soup – not one made with cream.

Check menus for "healthy" symbols. Many restaurants today are trying to accommodate patrons who are looking for simpler, healthier dishes. These are noted (sometimes with their calorie counts and other nutritional information) right on the menu. Check out the restaurant's website ahead of time to see if they offer healthier choices on the menu.

Search out restaurants that offer lighter fare. When choosing a restaurant, search online at www.healthydiningfinder.com or www.mobile.healthyout.com.

Share your meal or take half home. Restaurant portions are generally larger than what is recommended as a healthy serving size. Some places charge a fee for sharing a dish, but it may be worth it. If you don't want to pay extra, take the other half home to enjoy for lunch or dinner the next day.

Don't worry about getting your money's worth. Thinking this way could be your downfall. Eating out is about being with people and having a good time. If it's value you want, you'll get that with home-cooked meals. Eating in is good for the pocketbook, but eating out is good for the soul.

If you slip up, don't despair. When you do eat out, try to be extra vigilant, but if you do slip up, simply be sure to eat healthy the rest of the day or the next day.

Don't pass up the wine. If you drink, feel free to have a glass of red wine with dinner – but make it your only glass of the day. Otherwise, stick to still or sparkling water and lemon or unsweetened iced tea.

Yes, you can have dessert. A decaffeinated cappuccino or a cup of hot tea, especially green tea, can double as a dessert, and fresh fruit is always a sweet and perfect end to a good meal. More and more people are opting to order one dessert for every four to six people at the table, so everyone gets a forkful of delicious pie or cake or a spoonful (or maybe two) of ice cream. If there are only two of you dining, stick with the coffee and fruit, unless you're able to leave some of the dessert on the plate!

Holiday Eating

There's no doubt about it, holidays (especially those that focus on food) and vacations are dangerous to those trying to control what they eat. Holidays are the most difficult, because so many foods we associate with celebrations are filled with the very ingredients we are working to avoid. For some of us, there may be the added stress and tension of dealing with relatives. It's easy to revert back to old habits and lose yourself in food, especially when holiday dishes are probably childhood favorites and relatives are making sure you taste every one of them.

Be it Thanksgiving, Christmas, a Passover seder or a Fourth of July barbecue, those holiday foods are abundant in calories. But if you apply the rules you learned earlier in this book and in this chapter, you will get through the holidays without a problem.

Exercise can fall to the bottom of the list during holidays. If that happens, you won't be burning as many calories as usual. If possible, try to add additional steps to your day, or sneak in an extra exercise class. If that is not possible, be extra-vigilant when it comes to portion size. Eat less now, work less later.

If you are the cook, make this the time to prepare old favorites in healthier ways, cut down on the sugar, reduce the fat and salt, use the cooking techniques we talked about earlier and make sure there's a big salad and lots of vegetables on the menu!

If it's potluck, this is your chance to bring a healthy dish that you know you can eat.

Above all, the holidays are for enjoying the company of your family and friends. You may not lose weight during this time, but stay as active as you can because that will decrease your appetite, lower your stress and increase your metabolism. Your holiday goal is not to lose weight – it's not to gain any!

Vacations

When it comes to maintaining a healthy eating and exercise plan, vacations can be challenging, because every meal is essentially a restaurant meal. Even if you spend your vacation visiting friends, you may be eating out a lot or tempted with special meals and treats that your host prepared especially for you. But there are alternatives to eating everything that is put in front of you, including foods that are presented as a mouth-watering buffet.

And it's not just vacation eating that can be unhealthy. Simply traveling to or from your destination can be fraught with temptation. When you leave the house, be sure to take along healthy snacks that you enjoy and that travel well.

Everything you've learned about healthy eating and dining out applies to eating on vacation, so we won't repeat it here. But the main rule to remember is that being on vacation is no reason to ignore healthy eating habits. You don't want to undo weeks or months of effort in just a week or two! Below are some ideas on how to avoid the pitfalls you'll encounter when traveling.

Road Trips

When you travel by car, avoid roadside restaurants. Instead, pack a cooler of sandwiches, beverages and healthy snacks and picnic along the way. Take a short walk before getting back in the car. Save your food stops for those great farm stands and choose lots of regional fruits and vegetables that are delicious to eat raw. Don't forget to stay hydrated – water is always a good choice.

If you run out of food and must eat out, you know what to do, and if you don't, then reread this chapter!

Foods and Snacks That Travel Well

Traveling presents special problems, because the available foods may not be the healthiest choices. So pack snacks and other more substantial foods in a cooler or insulated bag to keep you from becoming so hungry that you'll forget about making healthy choices.

Below are some suggestions for tasty, healthy and energizing "travel" foods:

- Peanut (or other nut – no added sugar or salt) butter sandwiches (try adding banana and apple slices)

- Unsalted nuts or pumpkin seeds

- Carrot sticks with hummus or salsa

- Cheese sticks with whole-grain crackers

- Whole fruit

When You Arrive at Your Destination

Your room will probably have a refrigerator, and if you are diabetic, most establishments will supply you with a small fridge for insulin storage if you request one; this will also give you safe storage for food and snacks. If not, you can keep food in your cooler or insulated bag now that you have access to an ice machine.

Take inventory of the snack foods you have left and restock with items like fresh fruit, yogurt, cheese, nuts, whole-grain bread and nut butter or whole-grain cereal and nonfat milk. You will have access to healthy food and you will also save money.

Breakfast on the Go

The Breakfast Buffet

Breakfast buffets present a challenge because they are loaded with foods each of which could constitute a breakfast on its own, or shouldn't be served at breakfast at all (like donuts). Our advice is to sample a few things that you wouldn't ordinarily eat at home, but the key word is "sample." One breakfast buffet slice of bacon or sausage won't jeopardize your health, but we understand the difficulty of being confronted with many selections and not being able to partake of them all. Below are strategies for making wise choices that will leave you feeling satisfied and not deprived:

- Eggs are always a good choice, including vegetable omelets (no cheese), ready-made scrambled, soft boiled, hard boiled or poached (skip the fried eggs).

- One slice of bacon, a small piece of ham or one link or sausage patty is fine.

- Oatmeal or bran cereal (with low-fat or fat-free milk) is always a good choice.

- Fresh fruit can be used to top your cereal or as a breakfast "dessert."

- One small whole-wheat roll, slice of bread or bran muffin is fine, but avoid the Danish, bagels, donuts, scones and biscuits.

The Fast-Food Breakfast

Ordering in a restaurant or diner gives you the latitude to get a breakfast that resembles what you would make for yourself at home, but fast-food establishments don't fit that bill. You will need to order within their menu. Some fast-food places do offer egg-white sandwiches cooked to order. At other places you may be able to order an egg on an English muffin or breakfast burrito. Skip the bacon, sausage, ham and home fries. If oatmeal is on the menu, be sure it's not presweetened or loaded with dried fruit and nuts (ask if you can add them yourself).

Beverages

- Coffee and tea (hot or iced) are good with a little sweetener and milk.

- Stay away from high-calorie, low-fiber juice, even if it comes with your meal. It's not worth it in terms of your health. You're better off drinking water.

Happy travels!

P: Partner with Your Doctor, Family and Friends

Partnerships are powerful. They impact every facet of our lives and have the potential to increase performance, perseverance and results. When it comes to being heart healthy, partnerships are extra important.

As you begin Week 4 of the Six S.T.E.P.S. in Six Weeks Program, you have already restocked your kitchen with healthy foods, you are choosing to move more every day, you are enjoying colorful plates of fruits and vegetables and better managing your relationship with salt and sugar. Congratulations! Now it's time to consider the importance of partnerships on your journey to heart health.

First: find a doctor you like and trust. How pleased are you with your current doctor, and how trusting are you? Your relationship with your doctor is of utmost importance in your quest to stay healthy and free of heart disease. Think of your doctor as your partner in health; like any successful partnership, this one needs a bond of trust and an open line of communication.

The Power of
the Doctor/Patient Bond

If you only go to the doctor when you are sick, we need you to rethink that strategy. We know it's easy to put off making a doctor's appointment because of the demands of your job and your family and other responsibilities. But remember that many people who suffer fatal heart attacks didn't even know they had heart disease. The best way to diagnose and treat heart problems and the medical issues that lead to heart attack is to be seen regularly by a doctor.

Your Annual Well-Woman Visit

The way to forge a true partnership with your physician is through an annual well-woman visit. This provides you with an opportunity to review your health concerns with your doctor. It also provides your doctor with an opportunity to learn about you, your family history and any recent changes in health status, as well as to perform or discuss with you appropriate screening measures. At your well-woman visit, your doctor will examine you for any signs of heart disease, and he or she will recommend steps you can take to reduce risk factors before complications arise. This may include cholesterol screening, blood pressure monitoring, body mass index assessment and other evaluations specifically designed to help assess your heart health. These steps are a great way to help lower your risk of heart attack or stroke, and also to give you some peace of mind.

The well-woman visit also allows your doctor to review and identify any other health concerns and to ensure that you have received necessary and appropriate preventive measures, such as flu, tetanus and pneumonia shots. At this visit, your doctor will evaluate your health needs based on several factors, including your age, family history and past health history, and may also recommend that you be screened for other health issues that are unique to women including mammograms for breast cancer, pap smears for cervical cancer, prenatal care and bone-mass measurements for osteoporosis, as well as gender-neutral screenings and services such as colon cancer screening, obesity screening and counseling and screening for behavioral health concerns.

Just as you prepared for each of the lifestyle changes outlined in the previous chapters, you need to get into the mindset of scheduling a yearly well-woman visit. If you are anxious about going to the doctor for any reason, a yearly checkup should help put those fears to rest because they can validate the positive changes you are making. What's more, a yearly well-woman visit can diagnose potential problems before they become serious.

If you still have doubts about the need for an annual well-woman visit, those of you with children will recall well-baby visits to the pediatrician. You took them to the doctor just to make sure everything was fine, because you cared about their health and well-being. We all see the dentist for regular checkups and cleaning, even if we don't have a toothache, in order to keep our teeth and gums healthy. We see the gynecologist for a pap smear or to schedule a mammogram. So it makes sense to add your medical doctor or internist to your schedule of annual visits. Early detection and treatment of many types of medical problems, including heart disease, save lives.

Finding a Doctor

If you don't have a primary care physician, now is the time to find one you like and trust. An emergency room visit is not a substitute for an annual physical. You need to partner with a doctor who will get to know you and your health history. To help, here are a few suggestions and guidelines to make your search easier:

- Ask family, friends and coworkers for a recommendation and make a list.

- Check the listing of participating physicians on your health insurance plan's website to see if any are on your recommended list.

- Be sure the physician accepts your insurance when you make the appointment. If you don't have insurance, make that clear when you call.

- Talk to coworkers who have the same insurance plan as you and ask for the name of their doctor, and if they have had a positive experience.

- Check the website of a local hospital or health organization to see if they accept your insurance and for a listing of the physicians who work there.

- Consider only physicians who are board certified (which means they have passed special training and testing requirements) for the specialties of family medicine or general internal medicine.

- Check the physician's office hours and location(s); convenience should play a role in your selection.

- Choose a physician of the sex you will be most comfortable with.

Take your time and do some research. Finding the right doctor is important to your future health. You are looking for a doctor who will be your partner for a very long time.

Changing Doctors

In order to stay healthy, you need to have a good relationship with your doctor. If you don't like a doctor for *any* reason – be it trust, personality or something you can't put your finger on – then find another one. When you don't like your doctor you are less likely to make an appointment to see him or her, so find someone you like and with whom you can establish a trusting relationship. And don't feel guilty if you have decided your doctor is not the right partner for you. It's not your fault. Find someone you trust and don't settle for less, no matter what.

If you do decide to change doctors, remember that your medical records belong to you. Be sure to complete any paperwork necessary to ensure an efficient transfer of records from your former doctor to your new doctor.

Making the Most out of the First Visit

For those of you who are changing doctors or seeing a primary care physician for the first time, you will want to make the most of that first visit. If you are nervous, you are not alone. It's common for patients to be nervous or anxious when seeing a doctor – especially on the first visit. If you would feel more comfortable, consider bringing a family member or friend to this initial visit.

You will want to optimize your time with your new doctor, so here's what you can do to make the most of it:

- Be on time or a few minutes early.

- Have your insurance cards and medical information handy. If you don't have insurance, make sure you have the name of the person you spoke to when you made your appointment.

- Bring your notebook/journal and a pen with you and make sure you have recorded the following information in a special section:

  - Every medication you take, including dosage and time of day taken. Be sure to include all over-the-counter medications, including botanicals, vitamins, minerals, aspirin, cold remedies and allergy medication. If you prefer, you can gather up all the bottles, put them in a bag and bring them with you.

  - Your family medical history. Make a detailed list of the illnesses that affected your parents, grandparents, aunts, uncles or siblings. Also list first-degree relatives who have passed away and indicate their age and cause of death.

  - Any allergies you have to drugs, food, animals, pollen and so on.

  - Your detailed medical history, including hospitalizations, surgeries and chronic conditions.

  - *All* your medical complaints, in detail, and the length of time each has bothered you, with a description of the pain or the problem – in your own words. If, for instance, you have been getting a stabbing pain in your right arm that moves down to your elbow, write down exactly that and say it in that way to the doctor. Don't try to hide or down-play anything that is bothering you – tell it like it is.

- Questions to ask the doctor at the end of your visit. (See the list of suggestions that follow.)

Use your journal to record everything that the doctor tells you, because it's impossible to remember everything that was said. In addition, *never* be afraid to ask the doctor to repeat information or to explain it again if you didn't understand or hear it the first time.

Your annual checkup tells you and your doctor so much more than the state of your health at that moment. An annual checkup enables the doctor to diagnose and head off potential problems based on the physical examination in conjunction with your list of concerns and complaints. When you have answers, you will have peace of mind.

Questions to Ask the Doctor

The following are suggestions for compiling your list of questions. Not only is it a good idea to ask the doctor questions about anything that concerns you at the end of the first visit, it's also a good idea to compile this type of list for *every* doctor's visit. This list is only to be used as a guideline; be sure to personalize it by adding your own questions and concerns.

- What is my risk of heart disease based on my evaluation?

- When do I schedule my next visit, and is there any further testing to be scheduled before my next visit?

- Do I have a cardiovascular condition? How serious is it? What caused it, and how do I best manage it?

- What kinds of choices are within my control to favorably impact my condition?

- Can any medications prescribed at this visit interact with food or the drugs I already take? What are the possible side effects? Should the medication be taken at a particular time of day? How long do I need to take it and why?

- Do I call the doctor or go to the emergency room if I feel sick or think I have a reaction to any medications?

- Are there any programs I can enroll in to help me lose weight, stop smoking, reduce stress or learn to prepare food in a healthier way?

- Who in the office can I call with simple questions? (See the following section.)

Who's Who in Today's Doctor's Office

Remember, you should always follow your doctor's instructions and take your medication as prescribed, and don't try to second-guess your treatment. If you have questions or you think different aspects of your health care are causing you to have problems, tell your doctor. Only you know how you feel, but it's your physician and the other professionals in your physician's office who can help you solve any problems.

There was a time when the only people in the doctor's office were the doctor, the receptionist and a nurse to take our blood pressure and pulse, but times have changed. The modern medical office employs a number of people with various degrees and qualifications. The following is a comprehensive list of the people you may find tending to your health needs, depending on the size of the practice.

The physician (MD or DO) is the person in the office with the most training and is the one in charge. Doctors have anywhere from three to seven years of training after medical school.

The nurse practitioner/clinical nurse specialist (NP/CNS) is a registered nurse with a master's or doctoral degree and 500 to 700 hours of direct patient care. The NP/CNS has acquired the knowledge and clinical competence to diagnose medical problems, prescribe medications, order treatments and perform advanced medical procedures. Depending on the state in which he or she is licensed, an NP/CNS may or may not work independently from a physician. The training of an NP/CNS strongly emphasizes disease prevention and health management.

The physician assistant (PA) is licensed to practice medicine as part of a team supervised by a physician. PAs can prescribe medication in some states, order treatments and lab tests and diagnose illnesses and injuries. Most have a master's degree in addition to 2,000 hours of training with patients as part of their schooling.

The registered nurse (RN) is licensed by the state. Although RNs administer medication, care for patients and administer some procedures, they do so under the direction and guidance of a physician.

Medical students spend time rotating through doctors' offices as part of their training, so you may not see the same one twice. These students interact with patients by taking medical histories and may assist the doctor, but they cannot prescribe medication or perform tests on their own.

The technician ("tech") is a medical professional who holds an associate's degree in clinical laboratory science and is qualified to draw blood and perform routine medical tests, among them EKGs and mammograms. The tests that techs perform are dictated by the specialty of the medical practice in which they work. Techs work under the supervision of a doctor.

Don't Forget the Dentist

Another important doctor in your life is your dentist. It is just as important to schedule and keep your regular cleaning appointments, because people who suffer from periodontal (gum) disease are almost twice as likely to suffer from coronary artery disease. The science points to the fact that bacteria in the mouth affects the heart by entering the bloodstream and attaching to fatty plaques in the heart's blood vessels, which contributes to clot formation. As you have learned, blood clots can obstruct normal blood flow and restrict the nutrients and oxygen required for the heart to function properly, which can lead to a heart attack. Another possibility is that the inflammation caused by periodontal disease increases plaque buildup (this is different from the plaque that forms on your teeth), which may contribute to the swelling of the arteries.

Periodontal disease can also worsen existing heart conditions. If you suffer from a heart condition, be sure to inform your dentist. Also let your cardiologist know when you are going to see the dentist because you will need to be evaluated to determine if your heart condition requires that you take antibiotics prior to your dental procedures (including cleanings).

It's important to practice good oral hygiene: Brush twice a day and floss every night. Don't forget to get your teeth cleaned at least once a year, but every six months is better.

Get to know your doctor, dentist and the other medical professionals in your life. They are there to help you.

The Importance of Friends and Family

Nothing can substitute for the love and support we get from our friends and family. They are there when we need them, sometimes without our ever having to ask, and we try to be there for them as well. But what you might not know is how important these individuals are when it comes to maintaining your health.

Women who seek out the help and support of their friends and family stay motivated and are more successful in achieving their goals. The more people you reach out to in your circle – family, friends, neighbors, church members – the better you will do. Of course, these people won't be around to reward you with praise every time you make a healthy food choice, cook your own meals instead of stopping for fast food or exercise instead of lounging around the house, but if others are aware of what you're doing, they are likely to notice, encourage and compliment you on the positive changes. Maybe you are lucky enough to have people within your circle who will follow your example and join you for regular walks and adopt the rules for healthy cooking (especially at holidays and family gatherings). This reaching out ensures your success and allows you to share what you've learned with others who will likely be very interested once they see the results in the form of a healthier, more fit you.

You first need to decide what type of support is best and then figure out who is suited to give you positive reinforcement or even join you. Don't be shy about enlisting different people for different behaviors. Your sister might not be the best influence when it comes to refusing dessert, but a friend or workmate might. Perhaps a neighbor instead of your spouse will be the one to join you for an evening walk, and you might even motivate each other.

Be sure to log your achievements in your journal and review your entries every week so you have proof of just how much you've progressed. When you reach a milestone, like a good blood pressure reading, stable blood sugar numbers, lower cholesterol level or even dropping a pound or two, reward yourself. You deserve it. Nothing motivates like success!

S: Sleep More, Stress Less and Savor Life

Getting enough sleep is essential for a healthy heart. Too little sleep disturbs the body's chemistry and can cause you to be tired, irritable, depressed and susceptible to weight gain, all of which can lead to health issues. For example, the hormone that regulates hunger is suppressed when we're tired, resulting in inactivity and overeating. Both of these things can lead to weight gain and other risks for heart disease, such as hypertension and diabetes.

We all need to get sufficient sleep *every night*. We know you're busy, you have family to take care of, problems on the job, housework – but if you deprive yourself of sleep you will shorten your life, and that is no exaggeration.

It doesn't matter if the reason you're not getting enough sleep is because you stay up too late or because you are unable to get to sleep or stay asleep. The end result is the same, and it is detrimental to your emotional and physical well-being.

In addition, if you suffer from depression, diabetes, high blood pressure, high cholesterol or other problems brought about by lack of sleep, those problems and the medications used to treat them can also lead to difficulty sleeping. So it is vital to make getting enough sleep a priority before you get caught up in an unhealthy cycle. If you are already experiencing these problems sleeping, our Six S.T.E.P.S. Program can help you overcome them.

Adequate Sleep = Heart Health

Consistently getting a good night's sleep is good for the brain and the heart. Sleep recharges, repairs and rejuvenates the body. Adequate sleep keeps the entire body functioning efficiently and looking good (yes, "beauty sleep" is real). Insufficient sleep makes us prone to accidents, bad moods and depression and less able to deal with the stressful situations that lead to the physical ailments that cause heart problems. It's ironic that when we're not feeling well, are stressed out or are pressed for time, we tend to get less sleep, even though that is when we actually need it the most. This chapter will help you understand and overcome common sleep issues. If you can't fall asleep or stay asleep, make this a top priority to discuss with your doctor. Your health truly depends on it.

Not getting enough sleep...

*   Interferes with glucose metabolism leading to insulin resistance which often leads to Type 2 diabetes

*   Affects production of growth hormones and stress hormones

*   Increases risk of high blood pressure

*   Makes it difficult to control emotions and stress

*   Leads to inability to concentrate and make competent decisions

- Influences the production of the hormone that regulates hunger

- Reduces physical activity, which reduces energy expenditure and leads to weight gain

- Increases LDL (bad) cholesterol and lowers HDL (good) cholesterol

- Interferes with metabolizing of some medications

The good news is that with some lifestyle changes you can get enough sleep and wake refreshed every morning. Read on.

How to Get That Full Night's Sleep

Developing good sleep habits is the best way to get a full night's sleep. Many people who complain of not being able to sleep don't really have a problem; they just need to modify the everyday behaviors that sabotage their ability to get restful sleep. The following lifestyle changes can make getting a full night's sleep a reality:

- Avoid stimulants like caffeine or nicotine within three hours of going to bed. Also know that caffeine consumed at any time of day can disrupt a night's sleep. Caffeine is found in soft drinks, iced tea and even chocolate, so rethink eating that evening chocolate bar or drinking that cup of hot chocolate before bed.

- Avoid alcohol within three hours of going to bed. Although alcohol may allow you to fall asleep more quickly, it reduces REM (rapid eye movement) sleep. REM happens about 90 minutes after we fall asleep, and is thought to be restorative. Disruptions in REM sleep may cause daytime drowsiness and poor concentration.

- Don't nap for more than 20 to 30 minutes (and not too late in the day).

- Soak up some rays. Daylight promotes melatonin production, which regulates sleep and mood. Either get outdoors every morning or afternoon, or get a full-spectrum light (to simulate sunlight) for your home or office.

- Stay active. Make sure to move around during the day and expend enough energy to tire yourself out so you're able to sleep at bedtime.

- Set regular waking times and bedtimes. Try to go to bed at the same time every night and get up at the same time every morning – even on weekends.

- Turn off your mind. Take time to unwind or practice a relaxing bedtime ritual that functions to separate waking time from sleeping time. Try reading a book, listening to soft music or just spending some quiet time alone, away from noise and bright lights and electronic devices.

- Put away electronic visual devices. Switch off computers, tablets and smartphones at least an hour before bedtime, because the light they emit activates the mind, which will keep you awake.

- Don't drink liquids too close to bedtime, as this can make you get up during the night to use the bathroom.

- Check your medications. Some high blood pressure medications, steroids, antidepressants, decongestants and other drugs can interfere with the quality of or ability to sleep. Discuss these issues with your doctor to see if the dosage timing can be changed, or if an appropriate substitute can be prescribed.

· Regulate bedroom temperature, lighting and noise level. It's best to sleep in a cool, dark, quiet room. Use eye shades, blackout curtains and/or foam earplugs if needed.

· Eat at least two hours before you go to bed and if you must eat something close to bedtime, make it light.

· Use your bed for sleeping and sex – *only*. Your bed is not the place to do work, homework or anything else that does not involve pleasure, rest or relaxation, ultimately ending in sleep.

· Replace an old mattress or pillow to make your bed more inviting and comfortable. You'll look forward to going to bed when it provides a luxurious end to a long day.

Keep a Sleep Log

Keeping a sleep log may help you to identify what is causing or contributing to your sleep issues.

· Keep track of medications, activities and events in your life to see what is causing the problem.

· Use a section in your notebook as a sleep log. Record the time you go to bed and the time you wake up. Note if you fell asleep right away or not, if and when you woke up during the night and why, and the total number of hours you were actually asleep.

· Note how you feel each morning when you wake up (refreshed, tired, feeling foggy, etc.) and note anything that kept you awake or disrupted your sleep, including troubling thoughts of work, family or friends, a disturbing dream or pain, trouble breathing, a restless pet, light from another room or a street lamp, noisy neighbors/family, etc.

- Make a note before bed of how much caffeine, alcohol or medications you took, what time you ate dinner, how long and what time of day you exercised, how long you were outdoors.

- Note if you felt sleepy during the day. If you took a nap, note the time, and for how long.

- Record your nightly bedtime routine (taking a shower, reading a book, meditating, checking your phone or email, etc.).

- Keep the log for at least a week, but longer is better, to help isolate what is interfering with your ability to have a good night's sleep.

- Share your sleep log with your doctor if your journal doesn't provide you with the answers you need and you are still at a loss as to why you cannot sleep.

Also use your journal to identify things that cause you stress and then follow the relaxation techniques we outline later in this chapter. Once you find a technique that works, practice it every day. It will give you the chance to unwind and get on with your day. Finally, if you cannot overcome sleeplessness or anxiety/stress, or are kept awake by an active mind, nightmares, sleepwalking, snoring, inability to breathe, pain or other physical problems, make it a priority to talk to your doctor.

Helpful Hints for Restless Nights

If you're one of the fortunate ones who doesn't often have trouble sleeping but has the occasional restless night (perhaps when there is something important happening the next day), try this. Get out of bed and out of the bedroom and do something relaxing and nonstimulating that will free your mind. Read a book, watch TV, listen to soft music, pet your cat, until you feel tired enough to go back to bed.

When You Need Help Getting to Sleep

This goes for everyone: Resist the urge to take an over-the-counter sleep aid and *never* "borrow" prescription medication from a friend or family member. Not only do you run the risk of a sleep medication interfering with medications you are already taking, but some can leave you feeling foggy the next day, which is the opposite of what you want or need. If you and your physician ultimately determine that you will benefit from taking a sleep medication, follow your doctor's instructions and use only as prescribed.

How Many Hours Is Enough?

We grew up learning that eight hours was the magic number, but in reality it varies from person to person. The average adult needs at least seven hours, but many women do best with eight hours or more – especially when recovering from an illness. The key to knowing if you've had enough sleep is if you wake refreshed each morning and ready to start your day.

Getting an adequate amount of rest also provides you with the foundation for being able to problem solve. Tackling problems head on means they get resolved and go away rather than sticking around and wearing you down. Problems that aren't resolved can create a vicious cycle of stress/sleeplessness/health problems that you cannot afford.

When you awake refreshed, you think clearly and won't be easily overwhelmed. You will stay in a better mood, keep your blood pressure in check and be better equipped to maintain a healthy diet.

The Power of Napping

Taking a nap can save the day! It doesn't matter whether it's a daily nap or an emergency nap – the rule is that even though a nap can rejuvenate you when you're feeling tired, it's not to be used as a substitute for a good night's sleep. If you nap because you can't sleep through the night, then you have a problem that might require professional help. However, when you need a nap, take a nap. It can be a lifesaver for the occasional sleepless night, when you know you are anticipating a late-night event or just because you feel like taking a nap on a lazy day.

A nap of 20 to 30 minutes is best for improving alertness and not waking with that groggy feeling. Make sure that you nap early in the afternoon so as not to interfere with your regular bedtime.

Stress Less and Savor Life More

Stress! Stress is a fact of modern life, and there's no way to avoid it completely. But before we denigrate stress altogether, let's remember that some types of stress are actually beneficial because they make us put pressure on ourselves to complete tasks and accomplish what we need to.

Understanding Stress

Stress comes from our body's activation of the "fight-or-flight" mode, which is our instinctive response to dealing with situations we find fearful. This response has helped us to survive through the ages. When the body is in fight-or-flight mode it secretes adrenaline and cortisol (stress hormone), which cause us to become hyper-aware and focused and ready to respond physically and mentally to whatever is coming our way. So stress in its purest form is not a bad thing. However, problems arise when the stress we experience crosses the line from helping us get through the day to preventing us from living a happy and productive life.

Stress, if not controlled, can lead to depression and anxiety and set the stage for unhealthy behaviors that lead to poor health. Overeating, excessive drinking and smoking lead to physical issues such as weight gain, diabetes and high blood pressure – all the major risk factors of heart disease. And this is just the tip of the iceberg! Stress can cause irritability, inability to sleep, loss of sense of humor, excessive worrying, physical aches and pains, forgetfulness, depression and other psychological problems. These are some of the most common, but we are sure you'll be able to name others.

What this means to your overall health is that just as you must control what you eat and how much exercise you get, it's equally important to manage stress and keep it at a healthy level.

Three Types of Stress

Here's how, on a very basic level, stress can lead to heart disease. High levels of stress cause the release of cortisol, causing the heart to beat faster, blood pressure to rise and blood sugar levels to increase. Elevated levels of cortisol lead to an accumulation of belly fat, increased appetite and a craving for unhealthy, high-calorie foods. Stress is also a factor in causing weight gain because people who are under stress tend to be sedentary. In addition some people turn to smoking or excessive drinking in an effort to feel better, and both are detrimental to your heart health.

According to the American Psychological Association, there are three different types of stress, each with its own characteristics and symptoms:

1. **Acute stress:** This type of stress comes from the demands and pressures of everyday life. For example, the fender-bender in the parking lot, the deadline you are rushing to meet or the coffee that you spilled on your blouse before an important presentation; small, everyday crises that we tend to confront, deal with and move past. Common symptoms of acute stress are irritability, muscular pain, stomach problems, rapid heart rate, sweaty palms and heart palpitations.

2. **Episodic acute stress:** This type of stress occurs in those who suffer acute stress on a consistent basis, often individuals who are described as "Type A" personalities, or

chronic worriers. Common symptoms of episodic acute stress are persistent headaches, chronic high blood pressure and erratic sleep patterns.

3. **Chronic stress:** This type of stress comes from the major problems involved with such issues as taking care of an ailing family member or dealing with your own health issues, not having a job or enough money and so on. Chronic stress doesn't go away at the end of the day.

How Stress Affects the Heart

Stress affects the heart by:

*   Increasing the heartbeat and causing the arteries to constrict, which decreases blood.

*   Increasing certain factors in the blood that can damage the arteries that supply blood and nutrients to the heart.

*   Making blood sticky and increasing the likelihood of forming an artery-clogging clot, which can lead to a heart attack.

*   Temporarily raising cholesterol levels, preventing the body from ridding itself of fat molecules.

*   Influencing cravings for salt, fat and sugar to counteract tension, all of which cause weight gain.

*   Raising the amount of the hormone cortisol, which is responsible for the accumulation of belly fat.

- Complicating diabetes, because insulin, which regulates blood glucose levels, is not able to function appropriately, which causes blood sugar levels to rise. Cortisol also increases blood sugar levels.

Stress Is Caused by "Stressors"

Anything that causes stress is called a stressor. Stressors can be minor hassles, minor or major lifestyle changes or a combination of both. Since every one of us has to deal with stress of some type, the key is to figure out if your stressor is serious enough to impact your health. Take a moment and think about your daily activities at home and work. Because any activity has the potential to cause stress, especially activities caused by physical or emotional changes or changes in daily routine, take an inventory of what is going on in your life. Granted, some new changes, although they may be stressful, are actually good for you and will eventually become routine. However, the stressors you need to be aware of are the ones that don't let up and tend to wear you down.

List in your notebook *any* stressors that may be affecting your well-being. The list below will help you to identify some, and there may be some you are experiencing that aren't included.

- Daily hassles (commuting, shopping, cooking, housekeeping, etc.)

- Work overload

- Starting a new job

- Losing a job

- Retirement

- Financial worries

- Legal problems

- Change of residence

- Death of a relative or friend

- Ending a romantic relationship

- Disagreements with family, friends or coworkers

The Warning Signs of Too Much Stress

If any of the stressors in your life cause any of the following problems, this is an indication that you need to slow down and learn how to disarm that stressor and its unhealthy influence. Depending on the severity, you may want to consult with your physician.

Below are some of the ways that excess stress can manifest itself:

Physical signs: dizziness, aches, pains and muscle spasms, grinding or clenching of teeth, headaches, indigestion, muscle tension, sleeplessness, racing heartbeat, ringing in the ears, sweaty palms, chronic tiredness, exhaustion, trembling or excessive weight loss or gain

Emotional signs: anxiety, crying, anger, depression, feeling of powerlessness, hopelessess or loneliness, mood swings, irritability, negative outlook, nervousness, sadness

Cognitive signs: inability to concentrate, loss of sense of humor or inability to laugh, forgetfulness or poor memory, constant worrying, difficulty making decisions, lack of creativity

Behavioral signs: overeating, compulsive eating or other eating disorders, excessive drinking, smoking or drug use, quick temper, impulsive actions, constantly criticizing others, frequent job changes, withdrawal from personal relationships or social situations

How to Dial Down the Stress

We have provided you with a lot of information regarding stress and its effects on your health. Once you identify your stressors you can better manage them, thereby lessening their toll on your health. Below are 12 ways to reduce stress; you should choose the ones that work for you. Like anything else, there is more than one fix for everyone or every problem, and trial and error will show you which works best. If you are experiencing chronic stress due to unemployment, illness or family dysfunction, these techniques may help with some of your symptoms, but more focused medical and behavioral treatment may also be indicated. Nevertheless, these techniques can still help you relax and calm your mind, thereby lessening the impact of stress on your health. Again, make sure you let your physician know if the stress is overwhelming and basic stress reduction techniques are not sufficiently helpful.

1. **Reach out and enjoy time with friends and family.** You don't have to go it alone! Develop a supportive circle of trusting people and you'll always have someone there to listen when you need to talk about what's bothering you

or you want to share some good news. If you're feeling lonely, call someone – sometimes you have to make the first move.

2. **Breathe deeply.** Learning how to breathe deeply instead of shallowly from your chest (the routine way) is an important step in managing stress. With deep breathing, you really fill up your lungs with air and then let it out slowly in a smooth, even, rhythmic way. This type of deep diaphragm breathing promotes a good exchange of oxygen coming into the lungs with the waste product carbon dioxide going out. It helps the body to relax by stopping the fight-or-flight response and also has the ability to release its own built-in painkillers. Check out some of the many websites that offer detailed information about relaxation techniques related to breathing exercises, such as www.webmd.com, www.drweil.com and www.health.harvard.edu.

3. **Stop feeling rushed.** Make sure you allow yourself the time you need to get to where you are going and to do what you need to do. By allowing yourself five to 10 minutes more time than you think you need to perform any task, you can take the pressure off yourself. It's amazing the difference this one small change can make in improving the quality of your life.

4. **Schedule wisely and make lists.** Take a look at your date book, and if there's no white space in it, build in rest stops between appointments, chores and trips. That includes weekends and holidays. Keep a running and up-to-date to-do list so nothing will take you by surprise.

5. **Stick to your schedule.** Nothing can make you more stressed than the demands on your time by others. You've made a schedule; now stick to it by learning to say no. Of course you need to be realistic and flexible, and there will be exceptions, but they should be just that – exceptions. Be creative with your time, figure out shortcuts and don't procrastinate. Do the big jobs when you're fresh and the less important things when you're tired and don't have much brainpower left. When you're organized you'll have more time to do the things that energize and de-stress.

6. **Declutter and organize your living space.** Trying to live and function in a cluttered and disorganized house or office can drain your energy and cause you additional stress. Think about the anxiety you feel when you can't find something in a hurry (or at all). The stress this causes is as real as the precious time it wastes. Declutter your life so it's easy to find what you need. Enlist family members to help, at the very least, or to pick up after themselves. Keeping ahead of the laundry pile falls into this category.

7. **Get moving/stretch.** Take a walk, stretch in the shower (hot water loosens the muscles) or move around in any way you can. A good stretch or exercise session releases stored tension and makes you feel more relaxed and energized, ready to handle whatever comes your way.

8. **Schedule time to do what gives you joy.** Perhaps it's reading, gardening, seeing friends, taking a bath, playing on the computer, watching TV or spending quiet time with a pet. Pare down your to-do list and carve out some time to go out to dinner, to a movie or with the girls. The point

is to take a break from your regular routine, so block out this time as the important appointment it is. If you have set aside time to knit every Thursday at noon, then on Wednesday evening be certain to have your yarn, pattern and the correct size needles ready and waiting. Think of it as your "prescription" for health. Look through your calendar; we're sure you'll find some time for yourself!

9. **Prioritize and delegate.** There are always tasks and chores that you can ask family, friends or coworkers to help you do. Of course, there are things that only you can do yourself, but the point is that you don't need to do it all, all the time. Understanding this will alleviate stress and guilt. For example, if you walk your child to school, maybe you can share this responsibility with another parent or parents. Chances are that they will welcome the free time it brings them, too. Learn to ask for help when you need it. You can also make your life simpler by taking some of those chores off your current to-do list. Just as you don't need to do everything yourself, you don't need to do everything at once.

10. **Learn when "good enough" is good enough.** Sometimes we need to learn to settle for a result that is acceptable rather than always pursuing perfection. For example, getting the family together for dinner is more important than serving the perfect meal. If that means stopping at the local delicatessen to pick up a salad rather than making a home-cooked meal, consider that good enough!

11. **Get enough sleep.** You won't be able to cope with the trials of daily living or, in fact, any particularly stressful situations if you're not well rested.

12. **Practice relaxation techniques including meditation, biofeedback and visualization.** These relaxation techniques have been proven to reduce anxiety and the severity of congestive heart failure and headaches as well as controlling blood pressure and may even help prevent heart attacks and strokes and lower adrenaline levels, which also helps the heart. There are many reputable websites that can help you learn these techniques, such as www.nimh.nih.gov, www.heart.org and www.mayoclinic.org.

Some Stress-Busting Activities

Sometimes we need to take time out from our already full, stressed-out lives and do something fun to relieve stress. When we feel happy, it's easier to tackle life's daily challenges. Women tend to put their own needs last, and consequently, things that make them happy can fall by the wayside. It's like being on a hamster wheel. Once it's going around it's hard to get off, but you must stop the wheel and set aside time for yourself. For example:

Get a hobby. We're sure you have things you've always wanted to do, learn or try, and now that you've scheduled the time, do it! Drawing or painting, cards and games, knitting, needlepoint, crocheting, crosswords and Sudoku are all great stress relievers. Gardening is also a great hobby, and it gets you outdoors. Remember, a hobby is *any activity* done in your leisure time that gives you enjoyment. That's its sole purpose!

Schedule "me" time. Maybe you don't want a hobby; maybe what you need is time for yourself to do nothing in particular. That's great; just make sure you do it. Take a long bath, call a friend on the phone, or meet someone for breakfast, lunch or dinner. Go to a movie alone, take a walk or read a book. Just make sure that it's something you enjoy, that it's a break from your regular routine and that doing it will make you feel good.

Listen to (or play) music. Listening to music reduces stress and improves mental and physical health. What's great about this activity is that you can do it any time, even while you're doing other things. Turn on the radio (get a waterproof one for the shower), listen to your iPhone or put on a favorite CD and absorb the positive energy that comes from listening to music. Music also complements other healthy lifestyle habits by adding a sense of peace, putting a spring into your step or stimulating your mind, so take your music on your morning walk or have it on in the background as you read or write in your journal or exercise or cook dinner. If you play an instrument, that's the perfect way to let the music work its magic.

Take time to laugh. Laughter is good for your health. We're not kidding. Read some jokes on the internet, call a friend, learn a joke, watch a funny movie... whatever it takes. Laughing actually causes healthy changes in the body. It relaxes the body, decreases production of stress hormones, produces antibodies to help boost the immune system, triggers the production of endorphins that reduce pain and protects against heart attack by improving blood flow. Laughing also helps us to bond with others. Follow our prescription and take advantage of this free medicine – at least once a day.

Reward yourself. We are talking about treating yourself to something special that doesn't necessarily cost money. For example, light some candles and take a long bath, enjoy a night out at the movies, have dinner with your girlfriends or buy yourself a small gift.

Maintain a Positive Attitude and Self-Esteem

More than anything, maintaining a positive attitude and good self-esteem gives you the wherewithal to view stress as a *challenge* rather than a *problem*. A positive attitude helps you when you encounter situations beyond your control, because it gives you the courage to accept and make the best of those situations. The following will help you better manage life's stress:

- **Stay calm.** Stop before you react. Breathe deeply. Rationally evaluate the choices available to you.

- **Give yourself a pep talk.** You can get through this situation.

- **Keep everything in perspective.** Consider possible solutions and act on one that is acceptable and feasible.

- **Prepare for the worst but hope for the best.** Never give up hope. Odds are that things will not be as bad as you imagine.

- **Appreciate the experience.** There is always a lesson to be learned. Anything you can learn, even from a difficult situation, can help you in the future.

- **Start each day with a healthy breakfast.** A well-balanced meal of protein, whole grains or complex carbs and fruit maintains blood sugar levels to give you the sustenance and strength to think clearly. If you need to eat on the run, instant oatmeal, granola, fruit and low-fat yogurt are good choices.

- **Take life one day at a time.** No matter how bad things seem, every day is a new day. Stress won't disappear from your life, but a positive attitude will help you manage it and prepare for what comes your way.

As you complete Week 5, it's important to recognize and appreciate the healthy changes you are making. Congratulations on your progress. Keep up the good work!

Permanent S.T.E.P.S. to Heart-Healthy Living

Now it's time to put into practice the heart-smart lifestyle changes you learned over the past five weeks. Remember those "small steps" mentioned at the beginning of this book? Integrating these new behaviors into your life will make them your new habits and your new habits will soon become permanent.

Back to Claudia

As we revisit Claudia, our 48-year-old banker, frequent business traveler and mother of two very active teenage girls, we are reminded that her symptoms of fatigue, palpitations, shortness of breath and general anxiety were actually all warning signs of a blockage in her coronary artery. Thankfully, Claudia and her doctors caught this in time and were able to address the problem by performing an emergency procedure in which they implanted a stent in Claudia's artery. However, the stent procedure is not where our story about Claudia ends, but rather where it begins. It is here that Claudia began following the Six S.T.E.P.S. Program in her journey to developing heart-healthy habits that will stay with her for a lifetime.

Claudia learned that, despite her busy schedule, her home must be stocked with healthy snack choices, whole fruits, vegetables and healthy fats. She engaged the help of her teenage daughters, who located several farmers' markets in the area and were willing to take turns doing the weekly shopping and stocking the pantry and the refrigerator with heart-healthy choices. In fact, they really enjoyed having the opportunity to take responsibility for choosing and buying their favorite fruits and vegetables, flavored waters and unsalted nuts and nut butters. They were also helping Mom.

Once Claudia and her daughters purged the house of processed foods and put in place a rotating shopping schedule for ensuring a well-stocked pantry, she was able to focus on her exercise routine. Even while traveling, she knew that if she couldn't get to a gym, she still had to incorporate 10,000 steps into her daily schedule. She purchased an inexpensive step tracker and began measuring all of her daily steps. She realized that there are countless opportunities to add steps to her day without significantly changing her travel routine, and she actually enjoyed the feeling of accomplishment and good health she was achieving.

Here is what she did: running in place for five to 10 minutes in her hotel room, taking the stairs instead of the elevator, walking to the office from her hotel or taking a short stroll after her lunch meeting, which all helped her to meet her goal. One of the unexpected benefits of incorporating additional steps into her business trip routine was that the added exercise actually helped Claudia sleep more soundly while she was away from home. And with the additional sleep came the benefit of feeling less stressed.

Claudia continued to follow our program, and to make small but meaningful changes to both her home life and her work and travel routine. She and her husband decided that after the girls' weekly Monday evening sporting events they would no longer stop at a fast-food restaurant for dinner. Instead, they would come home and have "meatless Mondays," where the whole family could participate in chopping vegetables and choosing favorite legumes for an entrée-sized dinner salad. They began to look forward to these meals, as it was a time for them to put cell phones, television programs and computers aside, participate in a family activity and discuss the events of the day.

Returning to her love of photography, Claudia started taking her camera on business trips. She managed to find 30 minutes to an hour during each trip to take photographs, which allowed her to relax and reduce her stress level. She shared her portfolio of photographs with her doctor, who couldn't help noticing how happy resuming her nearly forgotten hobby had made her. Her doctor recommended that she practice "mindfulness" to further reduce her stress level. Claudia found that by using simple breathing and meditation techniques, she was able to slow down and de-stress during those difficult times at home and at work.

Claudia's doctor also suggested that she join a support group where she would benefit from the shared experiences of other women with heart disease. Claudia took this advice and joined WomenHeart: The National Coalition for Women with Heart Disease (www.womenheart.org), where she met other women who shared their challenges and successes in dealing with heart disease.

Claudia is a success story. At her three-month followup visit, she and her doctor were thrilled to note the following: As a result of her adherence to the Six S.T.E.P.S. in Six Weeks Program, her blood pressure was finally in the normal range and she was able to lower the dose of her blood pressure medication.

On Your Way to Heart Health

Claudia's example demonstrates that it is possible to make simple changes to your life, even if you have a job, a family and a demanding travel schedule. Although these changes seem small, they are crucial to getting you on the road to health and overall wellness. You can make these changes gradually, but making them is essential if you are going to live a heart-smart life. Once you start seeing the benefits (and you will), it will become increasingly easy to maintain these new habits. These simple small steps will help you to arrive at a healthier lifestyle and become truly *heart smart*!

Week 6 is the time to review your successes and evaluate where you have opportunities for improvement. It's important to celebrate those successes and be proud of them. But you will also learn a lot from your failures when you identify what didn't work and understand why.

Looking back over the past weeks, think about your successes and challenges and record them in your notebook. Did you have a harder time with changing your eating habits than with exercise or managing stress? Was it easy for you to choose to eat healthier food? As you moved on to Week 2 and added exercise, perhaps you made great strides with your new exercise routine but had challenges maintaining that healthier eating routine. If you have had challenges, you are not alone! It is common for one aspect of the program to work better than another when taking on new lifestyle changes over a fairly short period of time. Your commitment to living a heart-smart life is a long-term commitment, and your journal will be a valuable tool to help you get there.

As Week Six comes to a close, it is time to congratulate yourself. You are well on your way to solidifying the new habits you've developed over the course of the past six weeks. So reward yourself with that new outfit, a short holiday or a day of complete relaxation and pampering. But remember, the true reward is that you have finally put yourself first and are living your optimal heart-smart life.

To paraphrase Aristotle:

"We are what we repeatedly do. Good health, then, is not an act but a habit."

Rx to Lower the Risk of Recurrence: Secondary Prevention

For Heart Attack Survivors

If you have survived a heart attack, you have a lot to be thankful for! Over the past two decades significant advances have been made in diagnosing and treating women with heart disease. The combination of awareness and treatment is estimated to save the lives of more than 300 women who suffer from all forms of heart disease *every day*. We call this secondary prevention.

If you have survived a heart attack, you may still be scared, confused or worried about making certain lifestyle changes and perhaps adding new medications to your daily routine. If you don't make changes in your life and address what put you at risk of heart attack in the first place, you are in danger of having another one. Now is the time to start over and follow the advice we have given you to stay on the road to good health.

This appendix provides information relevant to women who have already had a heart attack. (Even if you haven't suffered one yourself, you may wish to continue reading to help or support a friend or loved one who has.) After a heart attack, you may worry about resuming regular daily activities or adhering to the rules of healthy living. But there is nothing to worry about. You can do this if you focus on making small but consistent changes to the way you live.

Healing After Open-Heart Surgery

If your surgery left you with an incision on your chest along the breastbone (sternum), wait for the bone and skin to heal before you resume normal activities. This takes anywhere from six to 10 weeks. You will likely be seeing your heart surgeon for regular followups in the first two to three months after your operation, and the surgeon will inform you when your sternum has healed.

Even after the skin is healed and the breastbone has knitted completely, this area can remain sensitive for a while, so you may need to be creative in terms of your clothing, undergarments, sleeping position and routine activities of living, including sexual activity and positions. (See "Yes, Sex!" later in this section.) This is temporary. Once the breastbone is totally healed, these issues should not be of further concern. If you have any reservations, talk to your doctor.

The Importance of Cardiac Rehabilitation

Whether you had a heart attack, underwent a stent placement, had open heart surgery or discovered that your shortness of breath was related to heart failure, your doctor will likely recommend you enroll in a cardiac rehabilitation program. Cardiac rehab is designed specifically to help you recover after a heart procedure, heart attack or hospitalization, or even stop the progression of the disease after a new diagnosis of certain heart conditions. Cardiac rehab has been shown to decrease mortality rates, reduce symptoms of heart disease and decrease hospital readmissions.

Cardiac rehabilitation and other secondary prevention programs have been developed to protect against the recurrence of heart attacks through graduated physical activity and muscle training. This physical training along with education and counseling will provide you with a better understanding of your condition along with practical ways to eat healthier and manage stress, anger and depression – all common factors in heart disease. Cardiac rehab programs are especially valuable – and underused by women! A coordinated team of doctors, nurses and physical therapists runs these programs, many of which also offer the services of dieticians and behavioral health professionals, as well as access to integrative health modalities like yoga and tai chi.

Getting into a Cardiac Rehab Program

Referral to cardiac rehab should be discussed with your doctor at the time of your heart event. You may need to wait for several weeks to months before it is safe to begin, and you will likely require a stress test to assess your ideal exercise prescription. Rehab sessions are usually two to three times each week for a minimum of 12 weeks. The program will be customized for you and take into account your physical activity prior to your heart event, your degree of physical stamina and medical facts about your heart along with the findings from your stress test. Physical activity will be monitored initially to check your EKG, heart rate and blood pressure, along with any symptoms you may feel (such as chest pain, breathlessness or leg fatigue). Your program will gradually increase in intensity and duration of exercise while you are being monitored. This approach allows you to safely learn the ideal way for you to stay physically active in the future. The careful monitoring, too, has been shown to be an effective way to help women increase their confidence and minimize their fears about being active. You'll take away from this rehab experience the knowledge to help you understand the importance of staying active and the wherewithal to do it on your own after the program is finished.

More Than Just Exercise

Cardiac rehab programs also include nutritional education and access to behavioral health professionals and other programs to optimize recovery. For example, there may be group sessions for stress management or a one-on-one evaluation with a psychologist or psychiatrist, because new research has confirmed what we have suspected: that stress, depression and feelings of anger can increase the risk of heart disease recurrence.

Cardiac rehab programs also include help for stopping smoking, referrals to sleep programs for those with sleep disorders and social support from other women.

Yes, Sex!

Sex is a subject on the mind of every heart patient. Whether you have had open heart surgery or a heart attack, we're sure you are wondering when you can resume sexual activity – or even *if* you can. The good news is that sex, like any other physical activity, will again be part of your life. Unless your doctor tells you otherwise, you can resume sexual activity when you feel comfortable doing it. Start slowly, and if anything bothers you or you feel physically uncomfortable, stop – just as you would when doing any exercise or even when climbing stairs. And, just as with starting any new exercise, report any new or unusual symptoms, such as chest pain, palpitations or breathlessness, to your doctor.

After open heart surgery, be the less active partner and avoid placing any pressure on your chest or breastbone. Remember, this is temporary. You will know when you are ready to resume your normal sexual positions.

Communication with your partner is crucial. Discuss your feelings and fears before resuming your sex life. Your partner probably has the same concerns. Talk them out, work around them and do not let them evolve into a stressful situation. Sex should be fun and should relieve stress – not cause it.

The Links Between Depression, Anxiety and Heart Disease

Behavioral cardiology is a relatively new area of research focusing on better understanding the connection between our hearts and behavioral health. But one thing is for sure – if you are feeling sad, angry or anxious after your heart event, you are not alone. Studies now prove strong links between depression, anxiety and heart disease in women. Not only are women who are depressed twice as likely to have heart problems (even if they don't have any other risk factors), but women with coronary heart disease who are depressed are twice as likely to suffer a fatal heart attack. It's also true that depression makes it more difficult to control blood pressure, which is crucial to preventing a heart attack.

More than 50 percent of women say they suffer from depression, anxiety or both as a result of their heart disease, which helps explain why so few women actually make lifestyle changes after experiencing a heart event. If you are depressed or anxious, you are unlikely to have the incentive or energy to make the changes necessary to prevent another event, and this can also lead to nonadherence to prescribed medications or followup doctor appointments.

If you find yourself feeling this way, do not suffer in silence. Call your doctor as soon as possible. When you are recuperating from a heart attack, your emotional health is as important as your physical health. So ask for help.

Depression and anxiety are medical conditions that are absolutely treatable and respond to a combination of medication and counseling. Do not try to fight them alone! Speak with your doctor about your symptoms, which may include anger, sadness, anxiety, lack of interest in pleasurable activities or significant changes in sleeping or eating patterns. This will be the first step toward getting your life back on track.

Even if you don't feel up to it, try to reach out to your friends and family. Stay in touch with a phone call or a note and maintain your social contacts. Having a strong support system improves survival in depressed women with heart disease. Your well-being and optimal recuperation depend on it. Help is available – but you need to ask for it.

Where to Get Help

Talk to your friends and family about heart disease. Explain to them what it is and talk about what you are going through. Some of the lifestyle changes you will be making will be easier if you have others understanding and participating with you. Collect brochures at the doctor's office, request information from the American Heart Association (www.heart.org) or WomenHeart (www.womenheart.org) about living with and coping with heart disease and share with those close to you. That way they will know what you are experiencing and how they can be helpful in your recovery.

Get professional help. Reach out to your doctor or other clinicians for a referral or recommendation that is right for you.

Check out support groups. Sometimes it helps to talk to others who are experiencing the same thing you are, and support groups can help you connect with other women who suffer from heart disease. Your doctor will be able to suggest those in your area.

Take medication as prescribed. If your doctor has prescribed antidepressants, always take them as prescribed. Remember that, in general, these medications do not work immediately but may take several weeks for optimal effect. For the majority of women it is the combination of counseling and medication that is most effective in fighting depression.

Exercise

Maintaining an exercise program is important in warding off heart disease, and it's equally important in preventing a second heart attack. Reread Week 2 of the Six S.T.E.P.S. in

Six Weeks Program and get moving every day. If you have concerns because of your heart attack or recovery from surgery and you aren't sure about how much to exercise or what types of exercise you should be doing, talk to your doctor about cardiac rehab. Your insurance may even cover it. With rehab, you will gain the confidence you need to get more physically active and have the added benefit of meeting others who are fighting the same medical issues. Statistics show that women not only benefit greatly from cardiac rehabilitation but also go on to have a better quality of life than before their heart attack.

It's worth repeating that it's never too late to start being more physically active. If you don't know where to start, refer back to Week 2 of the program for some guidelines. You don't need to join a gym, but at the very least, take a short daily walk and then walk longer and longer distances or perhaps go a bit faster as you get stronger. Walking is great exercise because it's aerobic and increases your heart rate, which has been shown to decrease the incidence of heart disease and stroke. Brisk walking has further been shown to decrease incidence of a heart attack and death from heart disease in women. If you prefer other types of aerobic exercise, like swimming, jogging, running and bicycling, great. Just check with your doctor before you start.

The bottom line is that physical activity keeps your heart and your bones healthy and strong, so *get moving*!

Take Your Medications

Be sure you are clear about *all* of the medications you are taking. This means knowing the name of every one, the dosage, the side effects and the proper time of day to take them. Properly taking the medications prescribed by your doctor can make a huge difference in your overall health and your ability to recuperate and prevent a second attack. If you have concerns about any of your prescriptions, talk to your doctor or pharmacist, and never stop taking any of them on your own without consulting your doctor. It can actually be dangerous to stop some medications abruptly. If you think you are having side effects from one or more of your meds, be sure to report these concerns to your doctor immediately. If the cost of your medications is an issue, mention this as well; there are often less expensive alternatives that your doctor can prescribe.

Aspirin

Studies show that for women who have had a heart attack, low-dose aspirin (81 mg) taken daily helps to lower the risk of having another one with the added benefit of preventing stroke. Aspirin also helps keep the arteries open in women who have had heart bypass or other procedures, such as coronary angioplasty. Taking aspirin regularly is particularly important if you had a stent placed after a heart attack; you should never stop taking it unless you are told to do so by your cardiologist. For some people, taking aspirin can have risks, especially if you have had serious bleeding in the past, so be sure to tell your doctor if this pertains to you.

Be careful not to confuse aspirin with other common over-the-counter pain-relieving products such as acetaminophen (Tylenol), ibuprofen (Advil, Motrin) or naproxen sodium (Aleve). These products are all effective for treating pain and fever, but only aspirin has been demonstrated to be beneficial

in preventing stroke or recurrent heart attack. If you are taking aspirin, do not take any of the above medications unless
your doctor approves. Always remember to tell your doctor
about all medications you take, even those that are over the
counter.

Birth Control Pills and Hormone Replacement Therapy (HRT)

The American Heart Association does *not* recommend that
HRT be given to prevent heart disease; it *does* recommend
that *any* woman who smokes, has heart disease or high blood
pressure or has suffered a stroke should *not take hormones.*

If you were taking HRT by mouth at the time of your heart
event, talk with your doctor about how to safely discontinue
use. Do not stop on your own or all at once. Topical estro-
gens, on the other hand, can be used even by many women
with heart disease to decrease symptoms of vaginal dryness,
but their use should be discussed with your doctor.

See the Dentist Regularly

Gum disease (gingivitis and periodontal disease) can make
you almost twice as likely to suffer from coronary artery disease. This may be because there is increased inflammation
from even mild periodontal disease or because bacteria in
the mouth enter the bloodstream and worsen the plaque
growing on the artery walls.

What's more, active gum disease can worsen an existing heart
condition by causing infective endocarditis. If your dentist
and cardiologist determine your heart problem puts you at
risk, then one of them will prescribe antibiotics for you to

take before all dental procedures. Be sure to take these anti-biotics as prescribed before every visit to a dentist, even for simple teeth cleanings.

Protect your heart by practicing good oral hygiene. Brush twice a day and floss every night before bed. Also make sure to have your teeth cleaned regularly, one to four times a year, as prescribed by your dentist.

Choose to Be Happy

When we feel good we are happy and optimistic about the future. If you don't feel this way most days or if you often wake up stressed out or worried, your health can be affected. Although some of us are naturally more happy or optimistic, we can all choose to be happier. The science of happiness has received a great deal of attention over the past decade, and we know that there are skills we can practice to lead toward living a happier and more optimistic life.

Of course we all have our off days, weeks and even months, but if you feel stressed, sad or pessimistic about the future, then you need to do something. Start with reaching out to friends, family and perhaps your doctor.

Don't assume the worst. You may just need a little emotional or psychological tune-up. Maybe it's time to resume a hobby that once gave you joy. Get out of the house and enjoy a movie, go to dinner, listen to some music. See some friends. Do anything you can to bring joy into your life. Perhaps what you need to do is knock a few things off your to-do list and have more time for yourself. Even having an extra 10 minutes a day to do absolutely nothing can be a help. It is just as important to make time for doing the activities that bring you joy as it is to identify, minimize or remove the stressors that make you unhappy.

Remember, as with all other lifestyle changes, it is not an all-or-nothing proposition. Some things that are stressful simply cannot be avoided, just as most of us are not able to enjoy endless leisure activities. But the important thing is to give yourself the choice to be happier by changing what you can.

Trust Your Intuition

We have heard many women say that they had a sense that something just wasn't right before they suffered a heart attack. There is something to that. If you suspect something isn't as it should be, trust your gut instinct – your woman's intuition. We have been around a long time, have seen enough patients and heard enough stories to know that acting on a strong hunch can be a lifesaver. Also, don't be afraid to get a second or even a third opinion if you feel any doctor is not taking your complaint seriously or minimizing your symptoms. If you continue to feel something's not right, find a doctor who will listen and will be responsive to your concerns.

Strength and Flexibility Exercises

Before beginning any strength and flexibility routine, you should consult with your physician. Once you are ready to begin your strength and flexibility training, you can use the following information as a general guide to get you started.

Flexibility Exercises

Do each stretching exercise three to five times at each session. Slowly stretch into the desired position, as far as possible without pain, and hold the stretch for 10 to 30 seconds. Relax, breathe, then repeat, trying to stretch farther. Here are eight flexibility exercises to get you started:

1. Neck stretch

2. Shoulder and upper arm stretch

3. Upper body stretch

4. Back-of-leg stretch

5. Thigh stretch

6. Hip stretch

7. Lower back stretch

8. Calf stretch

Neck Stretch

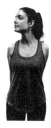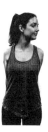

1. Stand or sit in a sturdy chair.

2. Keep your feet flat on the floor, shoulder width apart.

3. Slowly turn your head to the right until you feel a slight stretch. Be careful not to tip or tilt your head forward or backward, but hold it in a comfortable position.

4. Hold the position for 10 to 30 seconds.

5. Turn your head to the left and hold the position for 10 to 30 seconds.

6. Repeat at least three to five times.

Shoulder and Upper Arm Stretch

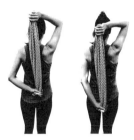

1. Stand with your feet shoulder width apart.

2. Hold one end of a towel in your right hand.

3. Raise and bend your right arm to drape the towel down your back. Keep your right arm in this position and continue holding on to the towel.

4. Reach behind your lower back and grasp the towel with your left hand.

5. To stretch your right shoulder, pull the towel down with your left hand. Stop when you feel a stretch or slight discomfort in your right shoulder.

6. Repeat at least three to five times.

7. Reverse positions and repeat at least three to five times.

Upper Body Stretch

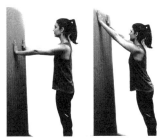

1. Stand facing a wall slightly farther than arms' length away, feet shoulder width apart.

2. Lean your body forward and put your palms flat against the wall at shoulder height and shoulder width apart.

3. Keeping your back straight, slowly walk your hands up the wall until your arms are above your head.

4. Hold your arms overhead for about 10 to 30 seconds.

5. Slowly walk your hands back down.

6. Repeat at least three to five times.

Back-of-Leg Stretch

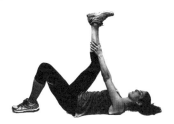

1. Lie on your back with your left knee bent and your left foot flat on the floor.

2. Raise your right leg, keeping your knee slightly bent.

3. Reach up and grasp your right leg with both hands, keeping your head and shoulders flat on the floor.

4. Gently pull your right leg toward your body until you feel a stretch in the back of your leg.

5. Hold position for 10 to 30 seconds.

6. Repeat at least three to five times.

7. Repeat at least three to five times with left leg.

Thigh Stretch

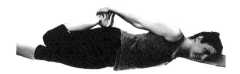

1. Lie on your side with your legs straight and your knees together.

2. Rest your head on your arm.

3. Bend your top knee and reach back and grab the top of your foot. If you can't reach your foot, loop a resistance band, belt or towel over your foot and hold both ends.

4. Gently pull your leg until you feel a stretch in your thigh.

5. Hold position for 10 to 30 seconds.

6. Repeat at least three to five times.

7. Repeat at least three to five times with your other leg.

Hip Stretch

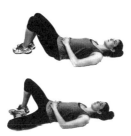

1. Lie on your back with your legs together, knees bent and feet flat on the floor. Try to keep both shoulders on the floor throughout the stretch.

2. Slowly lower one knee by opening out to the side as far as you comfortably can. Keep your feet close together and try not to move the other leg.

3. Hold position for 10 to 30 seconds.

4. Bring knee back up slowly.

5. Repeat at least three to five times.

6. Repeat at least three to five times with your other leg.

Lower Back Stretch

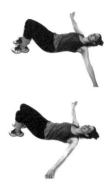

1. Lie on your back with your legs together, knees bent and feet flat on the floor. Try to keep both arms and shoulders flat on the floor throughout the stretch.

2. Keeping your knees bent and together, slowly lower both legs to one side as far as you comfortably can.

3. Hold position for 10 to 30 seconds.

4. Bring your legs back up slowly and repeat toward the other side.

5. Continue alternating sides for at least three to five times on each side.

Calf Stretch

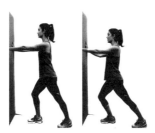

1. Stand facing a wall slightly farther than arms' length away, feet shoulder width apart.

2. Put your palms flat against the wall at shoulder height and shoulder width apart.

3. Step forward with your right leg and bend your right knee. Keeping both feet flat on the floor, bend your left knee slightly until you feel a stretch in your left calf muscle. It shouldn't feel uncomfortable. If you don't feel a stretch, bend your right knee until you do.

4. Hold position for 10 to 30 seconds and then return to the starting position.

5. Repeat with your left leg.

6. Continue alternating legs for at least three to five times each leg.

Strength-Training Exercises

Strength training builds muscle. When you begin your strength training, choose weights or a resistance level that allows you to do two sets of 10 repetitions. When that becomes too easy, increase the weight or resistance. With respect to weight-bearing exercises (push-ups, planks, squats, etc.), start with two sets of one or two repetitions and work your way up to two sets of 10.

Try to do strength-training exercises for all of your major muscle groups on two or more days per week for 30 minutes at a time, but don't exercise the same muscle group on any two days in a row.

The six strength-training exercises shown below target the upper and lower body.

Upper Body Exercises

1. Arm curls

2. Side arm raises

3. Chair dips

Lower Body Exercises

1. Back leg raises

2. Leg straightening exercises

3. Toe stands

Arm Curls

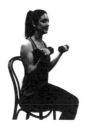

1. Stand or sit with your feet shoulder width apart.

2. Hold the weights straight down at your sides, palms facing forward. Breathe in slowly.

3. Breathe out as you slowly bend your elbows and lift the weights toward your chest. Keep your elbows at your sides.

4. Hold the position for one second.

5. Breathe in as you slowly lower your arms.

6. Repeat 10 to 15 times.

7. Rest, then repeat 10 to 15 more times.

Side Arm Raises

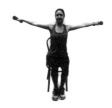

1. Stand or sit in a sturdy, armless chair.

2. Keep your feet flat on the floor, shoulder width apart.

3. Hold hand weights straight down at your sides with your palms facing inward.

4. Slowly breathe out as you raise both arms up to the side, shoulder height.

5. Hold the position for one second.

6. Breathe in as you slowly lower your arms to your sides.

7. Repeat 10 to 15 times.

8. Rest, then repeat 10 to 15 more times.

Chair Dips

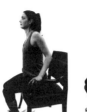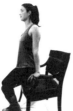

1. Sit in a sturdy chair with armrests with your feet flat on the floor, shoulder width apart.

2. Lean slightly forward; keep your back and shoulders straight.

3. Grasp the arms of the chair with your hands next to you. Breathe in slowly.

4. Breathe out and use your arms to push your body slowly off the chair.

5. Hold position for one second.

6. Breathe in as you slowly lower yourself back down.

7. Repeat 10 to 15 times.

8. Rest, then repeat 10 to 15 more times.

Back Leg Raises

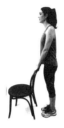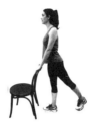

1. Hold onto the back of a sturdy chair or counter for balance. Breathe in slowly.

2. Breathe out and slowly lift one leg straight back without bending your knee or pointing your toes. Try not to lean forward. The leg you are standing on should be slightly bent.

3. Hold position for one second.

4. Breathe in as you slowly lower your leg.

5. Repeat 10 to 15 times.

6. Repeat 10 to 15 times with other leg.

7. Repeat 10 to 15 more times with each leg.

Leg Strengthening Exercises

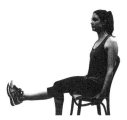

1. Sit in a sturdy chair with your back supported by the chair. Only the balls of your feet and your toes should rest on the floor.

2. Put a rolled bath towel at the edge of the chair under thighs for support.

3. Breathe in slowly.

4. Breathe out and slowly extend one leg in front of you as straight as possible, but don't lock your knee.

5. Flex foot to point toes toward the ceiling. Hold position for one second.

6. Breathe in as you slowly lower leg back down.

7. Repeat 10 to 15 times.

8. Repeat 10 to 15 times with other leg.

9. Repeat 10 to 15 more times with each leg.

Toe Stands

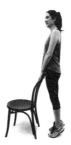

1. Stand behind a sturdy chair, feet shoulder width apart, holding on for balance. Breathe in slowly.

2. Breathe out and slowly stand on tiptoes, as high as possible.

3. Hold position for one second.

4. Breathe in as you slowly lower heels to the floor.

5. Repeat 10 to 15 times.

6. Rest, then repeat 10 to 15 more times.

As noted earlier, these exercises are provided as a general guide to get you started on an exercise routine. Depending on your level of fitness you may want to engage in a more challenging set of exercises. For a more comprehensive plan see Harvard Health publications at www.health.harvard.edu or the American Heart Association's website at www.healthyforgood.heart.org

There are also many videos and books to help you map out your own exercise routine, but we recommend *Mayo Clinic Fitness for Everybody*. This book contains 150 easy-to-follow illustrated exercises and is available online through www.amazon.com or www.bookstore.mayoclinic.com.

Common Heart Medications, Treatments and Tests

Once heart disease has developed, or in an effort to reduce your risk of developing heart disease when risk factors are present, there are several treatment options, beginning with various types of medications. Some medicines decrease the workload on the heart, while others reduce the chance of having a heart attack or dying suddenly. Still others prevent or delay the need for a special procedure, such as angioplasty or bypass surgery. Several types of medicine are commonly used.

Medications

ACEIs (angiotensin-converting enzyme inhibitors) help to lower blood pressure and reduce strain on your heart. They may also reduce the risk of a future heart attack and heart failure. Commonly used ACE inhibitors include: benazepril (Lotensin), captopril (Capoten), enalapril (Vasotec), lisinopril (Prinivil, Zestril) and ramipril (Altace).

ARBs (angiotensin receptor blocking agents) are similar to ACEIs in their indications for use and protective effects for those with hypertension, heart failure or even kidney disease.

ARBs are less likely to result in the side effect of a cough, which can be seen with ACEIs.

Anticoagulants help to prevent clots from forming in your arteries and blocking blood flow. In certain abnormal heart rhythms, they may be prescribed to decrease the risk of stroke. A commonly used anticoagulant is warfarin (Coumadin).

Novel oral anticoagulants are newer agents that are used for similar indications as traditional anticoagulants but do not require regular blood tests to monitor dosing. These include dabigatran (Pradaxa), apixaban (Eliquis) and rivaroxaban (Xarelto).

Aspirin and other antiplatelet agents help prevent clots from forming in your arteries and blocking blood flow. Aspirin may not be appropriate for some people, because it increases the risk of bleeding. Other antiplatelet agents that may be combined with aspirin include ticagrelor (Brilinta), prasugrel (Effient) and clopidagrel (Plavix).

Beta blockers slow your heart rate and lower your blood pressure to decrease the workload on your heart. They are used to relieve angina and may also reduce the risk of a future heart attack. They have also been found effective in treating heart failure. Commonly used beta blockers are atenolol (Tenormin), metoprolol (Lopressor), propranolol (Inderal) and carvedilol (Coreg).

Calcium channel blockers relax blood vessels and lower blood pressure, ease the heart's workload, help widen coronary arteries and relieve and control angina. They may also treat common causes of palpitations. Commonly used medications are amlodipine (Norvasc), verapamil and diltiazem (Cardizem).

Cholesterol-lowering medicines help to reduce your cholesterol to a doctor-recommended level. Commonly used cholesterol-lowering medications are the statins: simvastatin (Zocor), atorvastatin (Lipitor), rosuvastatin (Crestor) and pravastatin (Pravachol). Ezemitibe (Zetia) may be added to a statin for increased lipid lowering. Elevated triglycerides can be treated with gemfibrozil (Lopid) or fenofibrate (Tricor).

Long-acting nitrates are similar to nitroglycerin but are longer acting and can limit the occurrence of chest pain when used regularly over a long period. Commonly used nitrates are isosorbide dinitrate and nitroglycerin. A newer agent for those who continue to have chest pain despite the use of several medications is ranolazine (Ranexa).

A recent clinical research study showed that African-American patients with heart failure who take a fixed-dose combination of the medications isosorbide dinitrate and hydralazine (BiDil) had significantly decreased deaths from heart failure.

Nitroglycerin widens the coronary arteries, increasing blood flow to the heart muscle and relieving chest pain. Nitroglycerin sublingual (NTG-SL) tablets are small tablets that are placed under the tongue in the setting of acute chest pain.

Diuretics are used to lower blood pressure and can be helpful for patients with heart failure. They include furosemide (Lasix) and hydrochlorothiazide (HCTZ).

Invasive or Surgical Treatments

Surgery or a cardiac intervention, along with optimal medication use, may be indicated in certain clinical situations and may be more effective in managing symptoms and even in prolonging life. These treatments (angioplasty, stenting and bypass surgery) may be used to treat coronary artery disease if medications and lifestyle changes haven't improved symptoms, or if blockages are numerous and very severe.

Angioplasty opens blocked or narrowed coronary arteries, improving blood flow to the heart, relieving chest pain and possibly preventing a heart attack. Sometimes a device called a stent is placed in the artery to keep the artery open after the procedure.

During **coronary artery bypass surgery**, arteries or veins are taken from other places in your body to bypass narrowed coronary arteries. Bypass surgery can improve blood flow to the heart, relieve chest pain and prevent a heart attack.

Your doctor may prescribe **cardiac rehabilitation** for angina or after bypass surgery, angioplasty, a heart attack or worsening symptoms of heart failure. Cardiac rehab can help you recover faster, feel better and develop a healthier lifestyle. Almost everyone with coronary artery disease can benefit from cardiac rehab. Rehab usually includes exercise training and education about nutrition, stress management and other ways to live a healthier life.

Tests

Although we presented a heart disease "risk quiz" at the beginning of this book, there really isn't a standard heart disease test. If your doctor suspects heart disease, you will be asked about your medical history and your family's health. Next, the doctor will check to see if you have any risk factors and perform a physical exam. Based on the results of these preliminary procedures, your doctor may order an electro-cardiogram (EKG), an echocardiogram, a stress test or other diagnostic tests. These tests fall into two categories: noninva-sive and invasive.

Noninvasive Tests

Blood tests may be ordered by your doctor, including a fast-ing glucose test or a test called hemoglobin A1c (Hb A1c) to check your blood sugar level and a fasting lipoprotein pro-file to check your cholesterol levels. These tests can identify modifiable risk factors for cardiovascular disease.

A **chest x-ray** takes a picture of the organs and structures inside the chest, including the heart, lungs and blood vessels.

An **EKG** (electrocardiogram) measures the rate and regu-larity of your heartbeat, identifies prior heart attacks and checks for heart muscle thickening related to long-standing hypertension.

Stress tests are often used to diagnose when your heart is working harder and beating faster than when it is at rest. During exercise stress testing, your blood pressure and EKG readings are monitored while you walk or run on a treadmill or pedal a bicycle. For certain people, stress testing is com-bined with heart imaging.

Heart-imaging tests can be performed at rest to evaluate the structure of the heart, or they can be combined with exercise or medications that cause the heart to be "stressed" to answer questions about the presence of artery blockages or risk of heart attack.

Echocardiography uses sound waves to show the heart's structure, blood flow through the chambers and the strength of the heart muscle.

A **nuclear heart scan** uses a radioactive tracer and a special camera to evaluate the blood flow to the heart during exercise and at rest. A nuclear scan can find scar tissue indicating that a heart attack occurred.

A **CT scan of the heart** is a newer heart-imaging test that can be combined with a calcium artery score to provide noninvasive images of the coronary arteries and also to provide information about the beginnings of plaque formation in the arteries.

An **MRI of the heart** is also a newer heart-imaging test; it provides additional information about the heart's structure and function.

Invasive Tests

Cardiac catheterization (coronary angiography) can identify problems with the arteries of the heart. A thin plastic tube is passed through an artery in the groin or arm to reach the coronary arteries. A special dye is injected into the tube so x-rays can show whether there is any artery blockage or other heart problems.

Cardio-Oncology: The Need for Collaboration

In recent decades, we have seen a connection between cancer treatments and heart disease. Cancer therapies can increase a woman's risk of heart disease, due to the toxic nature of certain conventional cancer treatments as well as the "targeted" therapies, many of which have recognized or unrecognized cardiovascular side effects. For example, when a large volume of heart muscle is exposed to a high dose of radiation, problems can surface several years later in the heart and vascular system. For women who have been treated or are embarking on a treatment protocol for breast or other types of cancer, communication, collaboration and partnership between oncologist and cardiologist are vital.

The field of cardio-oncology is a subspecialty focused on identifying, preventing and treating heart-disease-related complications of cancer therapy, such as chemotherapy and radiation. The goal of the cardio-oncologist is to eliminate cardiac complications and maximize effective cancer treatment by:

- Prevention and early detection of cardiac complications

- Cardiovascular monitoring during anticancer therapy

- Treatment of heart disease that develops during chemo-therapy and radiation therapy

Women with preexisting cardiac risk factors such as obesity, diabetes, high blood pressure, family history, etc., are at an even greater risk of developing heart disease after cancer treatment. For those women, adhering to a heart-healthy lifestyle is critical. Women who are least likely to develop heart disease after cancer treatment are those who exercise regularly and are already at low risk based on their cholesterol, blood pressure and lipid profile.

Q & A About Heart Disease

Q. I was diagnosed with gestational diabetes during my second and third pregnancies, but this resolved after each delivery. Am I at risk for diabetes in the future? At risk for heart disease?

A. Recent research has shown that issues during pregnancy including high blood pressure, gestational diabetes, pre-eclampsia, eclampsia and babies born very small or very large are considered to be risk factors for future heart disease. Some have called these clinical conditions "failed stress tests" of pregnancy. They were included in the most recent guidelines on risk factors for heart disease in women. You should speak with your primary care doctor to see how to assess all your risks for heart disease and start early to minimize them. Women who have been diagnosed with gestational diabetes are also at significantly greater risk for developing Type 2 diabetes within five to 10 years after delivery.

Q. I recently had a heart attack, and I want to know when it is safe to return to sexual activity with my partner. Are there limitations?

A. Adjusting to life after a heart attack can be challenging, but we know that intimacy is an extremely important part of healing and living, so you should look at it as another physical activity you'll be resuming. The American Heart Association recently released recommendations about sex and heart disease. Unless your doctor tells you otherwise, you may resume sexual activity as soon as you feel comfortable. Always start slowly, and if you become uncomfortable, stop – just as you would when climbing stairs! If you are post-menopausal and suffer from vaginal dryness leading to painful intercourse, it is probably safe to use topical estrogen cream, but check with your doctor.

If you have had heart surgery and have an incision on your chest along the breastbone, you need to allow the bone and skin incision to heal. Sexual activity can be resumed slowly; you just need to be a bit more creative in terms of activities and positions, so take it easy. It's also best to be the less active partner during sex, and try to avoid placing pressure on your chest or breastbone.

Communication with your partner is crucial. Before resuming sexual activity, talk about your feelings and fears. Your partner most likely has the same fears and concerns that you do.

Q. I was diagnosed with lupus as a young adult. I have read about the link between inflammation and heart disease. Am I at higher risk because of my long-standing lupus?

A. Along with pregnancy-related conditions, rheumatologic diseases like lupus, rheumatoid arthritis and scleroderma are also risk factors for heart disease. These conditions are much more common in women than in men and have been shown to increase the risk of heart disease and stroke.

It is likely that the inflammatory abnormalities seen in these diseases cause inflammatory changes in blood vessels that lead to a higher risk of disease. Also, some of the medications used to treat these conditions, like steroids or prednisone, may increase the risk.

Q. I've recently heard about a cardiac condition called 'SCAD'. What is that, and is there any way to prevent or lessen the risk of developing SCAD?

A. SCAD, also known as Spontaneous Coronary Artery Dissection, is a rare, emergency condition that occurs when a tear forms in the one of the arteries in the heart. Although not exclusively seen in women, SCAD is more common in women who are pregnant or have recently given birth. Because SCAD generally occurs in otherwise healthy women, it can often be missed diagnostically. There is growing research related to SCAD in women, credited to the tireless work of a Women-Heart Champion with SCAD. The WomenHeart website (www.womenheart.org) can provide additional information about this condition.

Q. I thought "broken heart syndrome" was only something that happened in the movies. Is there really such a thing?

A. Broken heart syndrome, also known as Takotsubo Syndrome, is a condition that occurs as a result of a weakening of the left ventricle, the heart's main pumping chamber. This condition is usually related to severe emotional or physical stress, such as a sudden illness, the loss of a loved one, a serious accident or natural disaster. Symptoms include chest pain and shortness of breath and are often indistinguishable from those of a heart attack. The good news is that, once diagnosed and treated, it is usually reversible.

Q. Is it safe to take an aspirin a day to prevent heart disease?

A. If you've already had a heart attack, low-dose aspirin (81 mg daily) helps to lower the risk of having another one, and recent studies also have shown that low-dose aspirin prevents stroke in women. Aspirin also helps to keep arteries open if you have had a heart bypass or other artery-opening procedure such as coronary angioplasty. However, aspirin may be harmful for some people, especially those with gastrointestinal conditions like ulcer disease. Talk to your doctor about whether taking aspirin is right for you. Be sure not to confuse aspirin with other common pain-relieving products such as acetaminophen (Tylenol), ibuprofen (Advil, Motrin) and naproxen sodium (Aleve). For some women with known heart disease, nonsteroidal anti-inflammatory drugs like ibuprofen may in fact be harmful. Be sure to tell your doctor about all your medications, including vitamins and other over-the-counter agents.

Q. I know that stress isn't good for you, but are behavioral issues really related to heart disease?

A. We have long known that stress can be harmful, but there is more and more data that shows the harmful effects of stress, depression and even insufficient sleep in relation to heart disease. We also know that stress-reducing activities – yoga, mindfulness, cognitive behavior therapy – have a positive effect on heart health. And the importance of six to eight hours of sleep each night is clearly related to improved health.

Q. I heard that people with gum disease are at risk for heart disease. Is that true?

A. It's true. Researchers have found that people with gum disease are almost twice as likely to suffer from coronary artery disease as those without periodontal disease. There are several theories. First, many scientists believe that bacteria in the mouth can affect the heart by entering the bloodstream, attaching to fatty plaque in the heart blood vessels and contributing to clot formation. Coronary artery disease is characterized by a thickening of the walls of the coronary arteries due to the buildup of cholesterol and other fatty compounds, calcium and additional inflammatory substances. Blood clots can obstruct normal blood flow, restricting the amount of nutrients and oxygen required for the heart to function properly. This may lead to heart attacks. Another possibility is that the inflammation caused by periodontal disease increases plaque buildup, which may contribute to swelling of the arteries.

Periodontal disease also can worsen existing heart conditions. For example, patients at risk for infective endocarditis may require antibiotics before having any dental procedures. Your dentist and cardiologist will be able to determine whether your heart condition requires use of antibiotics prior to dental procedures. So practice good oral housekeeping: Brush twice a day and floss once every day. Have your teeth cleaned at least once a year (every six months is better).

Q. Do birth control pills or hormone replacement therapy (HRT) increase a woman's risk for heart disease?

A. For the vast majority of women, the use of birth control pills is safe. But women over the age of 35 or those with other cardiovascular risk factors, in particular, smoking, should speak with their physicians to weigh the risks and benefits of taking birth control pills.

Recent studies have shown that women who have gone through menopause and who have heart disease may have a higher risk of another cardiac problem – such as a heart attack – after starting HRT, at least in the short term. Women who have had a stroke have a higher risk of another stroke if they start HRT.

However, new studies show that many women may be able to use HRT beginning at menopause for a short period of time to minimize the vasomotor effects of no longer getting their periods. Also, topical estrogen can help with vaginal dryness.

Women should speak with their physicians to assess the risks versus benefits of HRT or other forms of estrogen replacement.

Q. Is it okay to take vitamins and herbs for heart problems?

A. When it comes to vitamins and herbs, it's always best to check with both your pharmacist and your doctor before adding them to your daily regimen. There is a common misconception that because a prescription isn't needed for vitamins and herbs, they're always safe to take. That is certainly not the case! All drugs, whether over the counter or prescription, can interact with each other – some in harmful ways. This is why communication with your doctor and pharmacist is crucial. It is important to bring along a written list of every drug, herb, supplement and vitamin you are taking. Drug interactions may not show up on the pharmacy computer if the list of what you are taking is incomplete.

But yes, you can take vitamins and herbal remedies, if your doctor and pharmacist know about them to ensure that there are not any side effects. Be sure to take your Rx and non-Rx medications list along whenever you go to a doctor, dentist, surgeon, nurse practitioner, nutritionist or hospital. Tell all of your providers what you are taking. It is your responsibility to do so. Only then can they provide the proper recommendations.

Q. I had open-heart surgery a few weeks ago. Why am I still so sad and tired?

A. Recent scientific studies have shown a strong link between depression and heart disease in women. Women who are depressed are twice as likely to suffer heart problems, even in the absence of other risk factors. Also, women with coronary heart disease are twice as likely to die if they show symptoms of depression. Depression also makes it harder to control blood pressure.

A very high percentage of women (more than half) say they suffer depression, anxiety or both as a result of heart disease.

But depression is absolutely treatable and responds to a combination of medication and counseling more than 90 percent of the time. In addition, strong social support improves survival in depressed women with heart disease.

An important component of cardiac rehab and secondary prevention programs is a focus on minimizing depression and anxiety after a heart event. Women are less likely to attend cardiac rehab programs and yet they are more likely to benefit from them! Ask your doctor how to find a cardiac rehab program in your area.

Depression can be conquered with a combination of social support, antidepressants and therapy. Collect brochures from your doctor's office and get information from the American Heart Association or WomenHeart about living and coping with heart disease. Share this information with your family and friends so they know what to expect and how they can help in your recovery from a heart attack or surgery.

Support groups are key. If you've done all that you feel you're capable of and you're still feeling depressed, seek out professional help. Don't hesitate to ask your doctor for a recommendation. Check the WomenHeart website, www.womenheart.org, for a group in your neighborhood.

Q. What about going to rehab or a gym after a heart attack? My doctor never mentioned it. Is it too late now?

A. It is never too late to start exercise, and you don't need to join a gym to get the benefits of exercise on the heart. If you've had a heart attack or coronary heart surgery, cardiac rehabilitation is of great benefit and is usually covered by insurance. So ask your doctor and sign up! Studies have shown that after heart attacks and coronary heart surgery, women benefit from cardiac rehabilitation and have a better quality of life. Cardiac rehab programs also include important programs on nutrition, stress management and other ways to lead a heart-healthy life after a cardiac event. These programs have been shown to decrease the risk of a second heart event.

Aerobic exercise, that is, exercise that increases your heart rate, such as walking, swimming, jogging and running, has been shown to decrease the incidence of heart disease and stroke. Brisk walking has been shown to decrease the incidence of heart attacks and death from heart disease in women. Therefore, a simple goal of incorporating walking into your daily life could help to prevent a heart attack.

Recent guidelines suggest 150 minutes of moderate-intensity activity each week or 75 minutes of high-intensity activity. Also, remember to do resistance training (light weights) and stretching regularly.

Q. I had breast cancer 10 years ago, and was treated with a combination of chemotherapy and radiation therapy. I have been cancer-free ever since, but I am wondering if this prior treatment has put my heart at risk.

A. Radiation therapy as well as other types of cancer treatment can present an increased risk of heart disease. If you are a cancer survivor who has had chemotherapy, radiation or any combination thereof, it is of the utmost importance to maintain a healthy lifestyle by following our Six S.T.E.P.S. Program. Exercise, maintaining a healthy weight, controlling blood pressure and preventing diabetes all positively impact the body's ability to compensate for the bodily stress of chemotherapy and radiation.

If you are about to embark upon a cancer treatment protocol, partnering with your oncologist and your cardiologist is essential to ensure the optimal combination and dose of therapies to maximize effectiveness in treating the cancer while also minimizing your risks of developing heart disease.

Q. I was recently diagnosed with lupus, an autoimmune disease. In assessing my risk factor profile, autoimmune diseases are included in the "modifiable" category. I don't understand this categorization, since this autoimmune disease will always be present and part of my overall health profile. Can you explain this?

A. As a general rule, risk factors that are considered modifiable are those that, once diagnosed (e.g., diabetes or autoimmune diseases), can have the inherent risk related to heart disease modified with appropriate treatment. Nonmodifiable risk factors such as family history or age cannot be "improved upon" in any way.

Reference Tools

Throughout this book we have included various suggestions regarding websites and organizations that are available to help you on your journey to living a heart-smart life. Below is a consolidated list of these references:

Heart-Health Organizations

American Heart Association (AHA): www.heart.org

WomenHeart: www.womenheart.org (for recipes, go to the "Resources" tab on the site)

American College of Cardiology (ACC): www.acc.org

Women's Heart Alliance: www.womensheartalliance.org

Smoking Cessation

National Cancer Institute Smoking Quit Line:
1-877-44U-QUIT

Additional Websites

Katz Institute for Women's Health:
www.northwell.edu/kiwh

Mayo Clinic: www.mayoclinic.org
                www.bookstore.mayoclinic.com

Harvard Health Publishing: www.health.harvard.edu

WebMD: www.webmd.com

National Heart, Lung and Blood Institute: www.nhlbi.nih.gov

AtheroSclerotic CardioVascular Disease Risk Estimator: www.tools.acc.org

Monterey Bay Aquarium Foundation: www.seafoodwatch.org (for information on sustainably sourced fish)

The People's Pharmacy: www.peoplespharmacy.com (for information on herbs and supplements go to "Home Remedies" tab on the site)

HealthyOut: mobile.healthyout.com (a mobile app for information on where to find healthy restaurant meals near you)

Portion Size Guidelines

FRUITS AND VEGETABLES
6 to 7 servings per day

1 cup of diced fruit

1 medium-size whole fruit or vegetable (such as a pear, orange, tomato, beet)

1 cup of cooked or raw vegetables

2 cups of raw or 1 cup of cooked leafy green vegetables

BEANS
at least 1 serving per day

½ cup cooked beans (can be added to soups or salads, or served as a side dish or main course)

GRAINS
5 to 6 servings per day

½ cup cooked pasta, brown rice or other grain

or 1 slice of whole grain bread

PROTEIN

2 ounces at breakfast (such as eggs, cottage cheese or yogurt)

4 ounces of lean protein at lunch and dinner

BEVERAGES

8 ounces or more per meal of water or other no-calorie drink

"Eyeballing" Portion Size

For ease when eating out, there are ways to eyeball the amount of food that constitutes one portion. Commit these basic measurements to memory or make a copy of these measuring guidelines and post them inside your kitchen cabinet or on the refrigerator door.

If measuring by cups and spoons:

1 cup = a baseball

½ cup = a light bulb

¼ cup = a large egg

1 ounce or 2 tablespoons = a golf ball

1 tablespoon = half a golf ball

If counting:

16 grapes = ½ cup

23 almonds = ¼ cup

24 pistachios = ¼ cup

1 cookie = 2 poker chips

1 brownie or piece of chocolate = dental floss package

12 baby carrots = 1 cup

12 strawberries = 1 cup

If measuring "by hand":

a closed fist = 1 cup/8 ounces/227 grams

an open palm (no fingers!) = 2-3 ounces/57 to 85 grams

a whole thumb = 1/8 cup/2 tablespoons /1 ounce /28 grams

a thumb tip = 1 teaspoon/4 grams

3 thumb tips = 1 tablespoon/12 grams

What ONE serving looks like:

3 ounces of lean protein (pork tenderloin, lamb, chicken, tofu) = a deck of cards

3 ounces of fish = a checkbook

1 ounce lunch meat or a pancake = a DVD/CD

1 white or sweet potato = a deck of cards

1 cup of diced fruit or raw or cooked vegetables = a baseball

1 medium fruit = a baseball

½ cup of cooked beans, pasta, rice, or grains = a light bulb

½ cup of frozen yogurt, ice cream, cottage cheese = a light bulb

1 tablespoon of butter, spread, mayo, salad dressing = a poker chip

1 ½ ounces of cheese = 3 stacked dice

2 tablespoons of nuts, dried fruit, hummus, peanut butter = a golf ball

1 muffin or biscuit = a hockey puck

1 bagel = a small tuna can

1 slice of bread = a deck of cards

3 cups of popcorn = 3 baseballs

Glossary

Aerobic exercise. Sustained exercise such as jogging, cycling or swimming that stimulates and strengthens the heart and lungs, thereby improving the body's utilization of oxygen.

Angina. Chest pain caused by a shortage of blood and oxygen to the heart.

Angioplasty. A procedure in which a device with a small balloon on the tip of a catheter is inserted into a blood vessel to open up a blocked area. Lasers may be used to help break up the plaque. Catheters also may have spinning wires or drill tips to clean out the plaque.

Anticoagulants. Drugs used to prevent the formation of blood clots.

Antigen. A substance recognized as foreign by the immune system.

Aorta. The main artery of the heart that begins at the opening of the heart's lower left chamber.

Arrhythmia. An abnormal heart rhythm.

Arteriogram. An x-ray of the arteries and veins that uses a special dye that can detect blockage or narrowing of the vessels. Also called an angiogram.

Artery. Blood vessel that carries blood from the heart to other parts of the body.

Atherosclerosis. A condition in which the artery walls thicken and narrow due to the buildup of cholesterol, restricting blood flow and leading to a heart attack or a stroke.

Atria. The heart's two upper chambers. The right atrium receives blood returning to the heart from the body. The left atrium receives oxygenated blood from the lungs.

Atrial fibrillation. Irregular beating of the left or right upper chamber of the heart when electrical signals are fired in a very fast and uncontrolled manner.

Atypical symptoms. Lacking the usual signs and symptoms that characterize a particular disease.

Autoimmune diseases. A varied group of illnesses that involve almost every human organ system, including the nervous, gastrointestinal and endocrine systems, as well as skin and other connective tissues, eyes, blood and blood vessels. The body's immune system becomes misdirected and attacks the very organs it was designed to protect. Autoimmune diseases include systemic lupus erythematosus, rheumatoid arthritis and Sjogren's syndrome. These diseases affect women three times more than men and are linked to an increased risk for heart disease.

Body mass index (BMI). A measure of body fat based on height and weight that applies to adult men and women. BMI categories: underweight = <18.5; normal weight = 18.5-24.9; overweight = 25-29.9; obese = 30 or greater.

Capillary. Thin-walled tube that carries blood between arteries and veins.

Cardiac arrest. A condition in which the heart stops beating.

Cardiac catheterization. An examination of the heart by threading a thin tube into a vein or artery and passing it into the heart to sample oxygen levels, measure pressure or take an x-ray.

Cardiac perfusion imaging. A noninvasive diagnostic procedure in which a small dose of radioactive fluid is injected into the bloodstream and collects in the wall of the heart, used to assess the heart's blood flow or heart attack damage.

Cardiology. A branch of medicine dealing with the heart and circulatory system.

Cardiomyopathy. A disease of the heart muscle in which the heart loses its ability to pump blood appropriately.

Cardiopulmonary resuscitation (CPR). a technique used in an emergency when someone's breathing has stopped or his or her heart has stopped beating.

Cardiovascular disease (CVD). Any abnormal condition of the heart or blood vessels, including coronary heart disease, stroke, congestive heart failure, peripheral vascular disease, congenital heart disease, endocarditis and many other conditions.

Cardiovascular. Pertaining to the heart and blood vessels.

Cardiovascular system. The heart, blood vessels and blood transported by the blood vessels.

Carotid arteries. The arteries located on either side of the neck that supply the brain with blood.

Carotid endarterectomy. Surgery used to remove fatty deposits from the carotid arteries.

Cholesterol. A waxy substance produced naturally by the liver that circulates in the blood and helps maintain tissues and cell membranes. Cholesterol is found throughout the body, including the nervous system, muscles, skin, liver, intestines and heart. Too much cholesterol can contribute to atherosclerosis and other forms of cardiovascular disease.

Computed tomography (CT or CAT scan). Detailed images of internal organs obtained by taking a series of x-ray images from different angles. Computer processing is used to create cross-sectional images or "slices" of the bones, blood vessels and soft tissues inside the body.

Coronary arteries. Blood vessels that receive oxygenated blood from the aorta and branch off into a network of smaller arteries that feed blood directly to the heart muscle.

Coronary artery disease (CAD). A condition caused by narrowed coronary arteries (atherosclerosis) that decreases the supply of blood to the heart (myocardial ischemia). Also known as ischemic heart disease.

Diabetes (diabetes mellitus). A disease that results in too much sugar in the blood.

Diaphragm. The dome-shaped muscle located at the bottom of the lungs, used in breathing.

Diastolic blood pressure. The lower number in a blood pressure reading that represents the pressure inside the arteries when the heart is filling up with blood between contractions.

Diuretic. A medication that increases the rate that urine is produced, promoting the excretion of salts and water.

Doppler ultrasound. A test that uses high-frequency sound waves to measure blood flow through the arteries and veins.

Echocardiography. A diagnostic technique using ultrasound waves to image the interior of the heart.

Eclampsia. Onset of seizures in a pregnant woman with pre-eclampsia (see definition below).

Electrocardiogram (EKG or ECG). A cardiovascular test that records the electrical impulses produced by the heart.

Heart attack. A condition that occurs when a section of the heart doesn't get enough oxygenated blood, caused by blockage of one or more of the coronary arteries.

Heart failure. Failure of the heart to pump blood with normal efficiency, causing inadequate blood flow to other organs such as the brain, liver and kidneys. This condition can be related to a cardiomyopathy and has previously been called congestive heart failure.

High-density lipoprotein (HDL). So-called good cholesterol containing mostly protein and less cholesterol and triglycerides; high levels are associated with lower risk of coronary heart disease.

Homocysteine. An amino acid that occurs normally in the body. In high levels, homocysteine may increase a person's chances of developing heart disease and stroke.

Hypertension. A chronic condition of abnormally high blood pressure.

Insulin resistance. A condition where the body is unable to properly respond to the insulin it makes. This can cause blood sugar to become elevated. Sometimes called prediabetes.

Ischemia. Decline in blood supply. Decreased blood flow to the heart, brain or other critical organs usually caused by narrowing or obstruction of an artery.

Lipids. Fatty substances (including cholesterol and triglycerides) that are found in blood and tissues.

Lipid profile. A series of blood tests used as a screening tool for abnormalities in cholesterol and triglycerides.

Lipoprotein. A particle found in blood that is a combination of lipid (fat) and protein.

Low-density lipoprotein (LDL). So-called bad cholesterol. High levels are associated with increased risk of coronary heart disease.

Menopause. Twelve months after menstruation ceases. The average age of menopause in the United States is 51 years.

Metabolic syndrome. Several conditions that, when they occur together, increase risk of heart disease, stroke and diabetes. These conditions include high blood pressure, high blood sugar, excess body fat surrounding the waist (apple shape) and abnormal triglyceride levels.

Monounsaturated fats. Considered the healthy fats. Liquid at room temperature and solid when chilled, these include such fats as olive, avocado and other nut oils.

Myocardial infarction. A blockage of blood flow to the heart muscle, causing damage to heart muscle cells. Also called heart attack.

Myocardial ischemia. Lack of oxygen-carrying blood in an area of heart tissue due to blocked coronary arteries. Myocardial ischemia can cause chest pain but it also can be painless. Without intervention, myocardial ischemia can lead to a heart attack.

Myocardium. The middle and thickest layer of heart muscle.

Nuclear stress test. Uses a radioactive tracer and a special camera to evaluate the blood flow to the heart during exercise and at rest. A nuclear scan can indicate whether there is scar tissue, meaning that a heart attack occurred.

Oxygen-free radicals. Toxic chemicals released during the process of cellular respiration and released in excessive amounts as a cell dies.

Pacemaker. An electrical device that controls the heartbeat and heart rhythm by emitting a series of electrical charges.

Palpitations. The feeling that the heart is fluttering, beating too fast or irregularly or skipping a beat.

Pericarditis. An inflammation or swelling of the membrane surrounding the heart.

Pericardium. The membrane surrounding the heart.

Polyunsaturated fats. Fat molecules that have more than one unsaturated carbon bond. Oils that contain polyunsaturated fats are typically liquid at room temperature but become solid when chilled. Polyunsaturated fats can help reduce blood cholesterol levels.

Peripheral artery disease. A condition where the arteries to the legs, arms and organs have narrowed. It can lead to pain and loss of function.

Plaque. Fatty substances including cholesterol, cellular waste products, calcium and fibrin (a clotting material in the blood) that build up in the lining of an artery.

Platelet. A colorless disk-shaped body in blood that aids clotting.

Prediabetes. A condition where blood sugar is high but not so high as to be classified as Type 2 diabetes. Sometimes referred to as impaired glucose tolerance.

Preeclampsia. A complication of pregnancy characterized by high blood pressure and signs of damage to another organ system, often the kidneys.

Prehypertension. A newly defined condition of having blood pressure between 120/80 and 139/89 mm Hg. This represents a warning sign that one is at higher risk of developing high blood pressure in the future.

Premature atrial contraction (PAC). Extra, abnormal heartbeats originating in the atrium that disrupt regular heart rhythm. PACs can feel like a flip-flop or skipped beat in the chest.

Premature ventricular contraction (PVC). Extra, abnormal heartbeats originating in the ventricle that disrupt regular heart rhythm. PVCs can feel like a flip-flop or skipped beat in the chest.

Protein. Amino acid compound that the body uses for growth and repair. Foods that supply the body with protein include animal products, grains, legumes and vegetables.

Pulmonary artery. Artery carrying deoxygenated blood from the heart to the lungs.

Pulse. Measure of the heart rate. A rhythmical throbbing of the arteries as blood is propelled through them, typically as felt in the wrists or neck.

Pulse foods. A pulse is an edible seed that grows in a pod. Pulses include all beans, peas and lentils. They are low-fat sources of protein, fiber, vitamins and minerals, and they count toward the recommended five daily portions of fruit and vegetables.

Saturated fat. Fat found in dairy products and meat; it contributes to raised cholesterol levels.

Silent ischemia. Ischemia without any pain or symptoms.

Spontaneous Coronary Artery Dissection (SCAD). A rare condition, where a sudden tear forms in the wall of a coronary artery. This results in ischemia, and can cause a heart attack, abnormal heart rhythm or death.

Statin. Any one of a class of drugs that reduce levels of LDL.

Stenosis. An abnormal narrowing of a blood vessel.

Stent. A tiny, expandable coil that is placed inside a blood vessel at the site of a blockage and then expanded to open up the blockage.

Stroke. Loss of muscle function, vision, sensation or speech caused by either a hemorrhage or an insufficient supply of blood to part of the brain. This may be due to narrowing of the arteries supplying blood to the brain. A hemorrhage may involve bleeding into the brain itself or the space around the brain.

Systolic blood pressure. The top number in a blood pressure reading, which is a measure of the pressure inside the arteries as the heart contracts.

Tachycardia. A rapid heartbeat. Sometimes this is a normal response to exercise, anxiety or fever. In some cases, the rapid heart rate is an abnormal response.

Takotsubo Cardiomyopathy. Also known as "broken heart syndrome", this is a temporary condition that occurs as a result acute weakening of the left ventricle, and is usually related to severe emotional or physical stress.

Total serum cholesterol. A combined measurement of a person's high-density lipoprotein (HDL), low-density lipoprotein (LDL) and triglycerides.

Triglycerides. Fats carried through the bloodstream to tissues. Most of the body's fat is stored in the form of triglycerides for later use. Triglycerides are obtained primarily from fat in foods.

Valve. A gate or door between two chambers of the heart or between a heart chamber and a blood vessel. When a heart valve is closed, no blood should pass through.

Vascular. Pertaining to the vessels that carry blood.

Ventricles. The two lower heart chambers. These chambers are responsible for pumping blood to the lungs (right ventricle) and body (left ventricle).

Ventricular tachycardia. Electrical signals in the ventricles that are fired in a very fast and uncontrolled manner, causing the heart to quiver rather than beat and pump blood. This can deteriorate to a more rapid, irregular rhythm sometimes referred to as ventricular fibrillation.

Acknowledgments

We had many partners in writing this book, and we want to take this opportunity to acknowledge and offer a heartfelt thanks to the village of women and men who inspired, assisted, and most importantly, cheered us on to the finish line.

To our remarkable, resilient patients, you are the reason we continue to be passionate about empowering women from all walks of life to take responsibility for their health and be their own best advocates. Your stories continue to be at the forefront of all we do. Your questions, concerns and requests for a simple plan for heart-healthy living were the catalysts for this book.

We want to acknowledge those without whom *Heart Smart for Women* would not have become a reality.

A sincere thanks to our co-writers, Sotiria Everett and Lori Russo. Sotiria successfully navigated the journey of many women in their quest for heart-healthy eating and developed a simple plan to guide them to heart-healthy food choices. Lori worked tirelessly to bring this book to completion. Her guidance, patience and expertise were invaluable.

Thanks to PJ Dempsey, for her enthusiasm, encouragement and guidance in getting us started. PJ, you ignited the fire and jump-started the writing of *Heart Smart for Women*.

Heartfelt gratitude to Jennifer Ashton, MD, for her thoughtful and insightful foreword, and to Hope Allen for her collaboration and expertise.

Thanks to our editor, Barbara Munson, for your insights and timely and superb feedback on the manuscript, as well as to the Onward team, Jeff Barasch, Justin Colby, Mary O'Connor and Thea Welch, for your guidance, feedback and expertise.

Our colleagues at the Katz Institute for Women's Health provided invaluable support and encouragement. Leslie Kang, Rosemarie Ennis, Rosagna Mancebo, Reva Gajer, Catherine Blotiau, Emilie Blotiau, Kaye-lani Brissett, Joan Bush, Lori Ginsberg, Bella Grossman, Marissa Licata, Kim McHugh, and Penny Stern, MD, we are truly blessed to work alongside all of you each and every day.

A world of thanks to our team members in the Center for Equity of Care, Barbara Milone, Michael Wright, Cynthia Lewin, Debbie DiMisa, Lori Loose, Elizabeth McCulloch, Fallon Williams, Marilyn Dienstag, Terry Tan, Elaine Ianazzi, Dorraine Russin, Samantha Rosario, Colleen Ruggiero and Shawn Crumpton.

Special thanks to Iris and Saul Katz, for their visionary approach to women's health and their commitment to empowering women to focus on prevention and wellness. We are honored to join you in this effort. This book would not have been possible without your foresight and strong support.

Thank you to Nanci and Larry Roth and the Roth Family Foundation for their generosity and support of the Women's Heart Health Program at Northwell. Through the program we are able to provide personalized care for the prevention, early detection and treatment of cardiovascular disease in women.

As long-time physicians at Northwell Health, we are indebted to our colleagues for embracing the need to see women's health differently. Thanks to our leadership team and colleagues: Michael Dowling, Mark Solazzo, Larry Smith, MD, David Battinelli, MD, Ralph Nappi, Kevin Beiner, Rachel Bond, MD, Jean Cacciabaudo, MD, Dennis Connors, Dennis Dowling, Donna Drummond, Victoria Faustini, Barbara Felker, Alice Fornari, Kathy Gallo, Rebecca Gordon, Evelina Grayver, MD, Cindy Grines, MD, Sonia Henry, MD, Jill Kalman, MD, Barry Kaplan, MD, Stanley Katz, MD Jeffrey Kraut, Brian Lally, Robert Lane, Winifred Mack, Phyllis McCready, Joe Moscola, Jason Naidich, MD, Ira Nash, MD, Laura Peabody, Portia Rindos, Angela Romano, MD, June Scarlett, Deborah Schiff, Joe Schulman, Varinder Singh, MD, Susan Somerville, Ramon Soto, Suzanne Steinbaum, DO, Eugene Tangney, Bessy Thangavelu, Chantal Weinhold, Maureen White, Abbey Wolf, MD, as well as the Katz Institute for Women's Health Clinical Steering Committee and the rest of our Northwell family.

Our friends at the American Heart Association have provided continued words of encouragement as well as the opportunity to meet many of the women who inspired us to write this book. Nancy Brown, Julie Roberts, Sue Flor, Kathy Munsch, Brooks Lancaster, Jaimie Racanelli, Heather Kinder, Kathy Kauffmann, Leslie Holland, Julie Del Barto and Larry Bloustein, you have been with us every step of the way.

A special thank you to our friends at WomenHeart for overseeing a comprehensive program of uniquely patient-centered initiatives, including Mary McGowan, Susan Campbell, Joyce Lenard and the physician members of the Scientific Advisory Council. In addition, we would like to thank our long-time champions, Ally Bunin, Michael Weamer and Helaine Baruch.

We are fortunate to have a continually expanding network of cardiology colleagues who are luminaries in their respective fields, collaborators and innovators on the journey to gender equity and women's heart health. We want to thank the incomparable Nanette Wenger, MD, our hero and mentor, and the champions of women's health, Drs. Holly Andersen, Sharonne Hayes, Noel Bairy Merz, Robert Bonow, Martha Gulati, Alice Jacobs, Gina Lundberg, Robin Miller, Rita Redberg, Leslee Shaw, Allison Spatz, Michelle Johnson, Annabelle Volgman, Mary (Minnow) Walsh, Malissa Wood, Virginia Miller and Ileana Pina.

It is difficult to find the right words with which to thank our families. Our parents, sisters, brothers, husbands and children have been there for us at every turn, and have inspired and encouraged us to make the concept for this book a reality.

To our remarkable, inspirational mothers and aunts, Jean Mieres, Harriet Rosen, Dimitra Tzakas, Rae Russo and Barbara Mieres, you have been our role models, our sounding boards and our best cheerleaders.

Most of all we wish to thank our husbands, Haskel Fleishaker, Mark Silverman, Andrew Everett and Barry Shpizner, and our children, Zoë Fleishaker, Max, Rebecca and Sarah Silverman, Dimitri, Matthew and Alexa Everett and Mark and Jeremy Shpizner. Without your encouragement, understanding, support and love we would not have been successful in this major and important accomplishment.

About the Authors

JENNIFER H. MIERES, MD, FACC, MASNC, FAHA, is a Professor of Cardiology and the Associate Dean of Faculty Affairs at the Donald and Barbara Zucker School of Medicine at Hofstra/Northwell, and Senior Vice President, Center for Equity of Care, and Chief Diversity and Inclusion Officer of Northwell Health. Dr. Mieres is a leading expert in the fields of nuclear cardiology, cardiovascular disease in women and patient-centered health care advocacy. As Senior Vice President of Northwell Health's Center for Equity of Care, she has oversight of the Katz Institute for Women's Health and several community outreach and community partnership programs.

A graduate of Bennington College and Boston University School of Medicine, she is a Fellow of the American Heart Association (AHA), American College of Cardiology (ACC) and American Society of Nuclear Cardiology (ASNC) and served as the first female President of the ASNC. She is board-certified in cardiovascular diseases and nuclear cardiology and is actively involved in clinical cardiovascular research.

Dr. Mieres is a leading advocate for health equity, women's health, patient-centered health care and medical education reform. Her research in women's cardiovascular health contributed to the nation's imaging guidelines for women. She was an executive producer of the documentary *A Woman's Heart* (2002), which was nominated for an Emmy for Best Documentary in the Health Science category at the 46th Annual New York Emmy Awards, as well as of a two-part documentary series aired nationally by

PBS, entitled *Rx: The Quiet Revolution* and *Rx: Doctors of Tomorrow* (2015).

Dr. Mieres co-authored *Heart Smart for Black Women and Latinas: A Five-Week Program for Living a Heart-Healthy Lifestyle* (2008) as well as over 60 scientific publications. A true patient and community advocate, Dr. Mieres serves as a national spokesperson for AHA's Go Red for Women movement, has served as chair of several national AHA committees and chaired the writing group on the AHA's first imaging guidelines for women with suspected heart disease. She is also a founding member of the Scientific Advisory Board for WomenHeart: The National Coalition for Women with Heart Disease.

Dr. Mieres has been recognized as a tireless force fostering diversity in medical education as well as eliminating disparities in the delivery of health care to the community. The Association of Black Cardiologists recently awarded her the Walter M. Booker Sr. Health Promotion Award. The American Heart Association has also recognized her for outstanding service as Regional President and for her significant volunteer contributions. Dr. Mieres has also received the National ACC's Women in Cardiology Mentoring Award; the Woman's Day Red Dress Award; the WomenHeart Wenger Award for Healthcare; and the New York State Governor's Award of Excellence.

Dr. Mieres is routinely called upon by national and local media for expert commentary and has been designated as a most credible voice in the health care industry.

Dr. Mieres currently lives in New York City with her husband, Dr. Haskel Fleishaker, and their daughter, Zoe.

STACEY E. ROSEN, MD, FACC, FACP, FAHA, is a Professor of Cardiology and Partners Council Professor of Women's Health at the Donald and Barbara Zucker School of Medicine at Hofstra/Northwell and Vice President, Women's Health, of the Katz Institute for Women's Health (KIWH).

At KIWH, Dr. Rosen oversees the development and coordination of a comprehensive and integrated approach to women's services at Northwell Health. KIWH focuses on the elimination of health care disparities through comprehensive clinical programs, gender-based research, community engagement and health literacy initiatives.

A graduate of the six-year medical program at Boston University School of Medicine, Dr. Rosen is board certified in Internal Medicine, Cardiology and Echocardiography and is a Fellow of the American College of Cardiology, the American College of Physicians, the American Heart Association and the American Society of Echocardiography.

Dr. Rosen has been a practicing cardiologist and echocardiographer for over 25 years and was the Associate Chairman of the Department of Cardiology and Director of the Cardiovascular Disease Fellowship Program at Northwell Health prior to joining KIWH.

Dr. Rosen has been a long-time volunteer for the AHA with leadership positions at the local, regional and national levels. She has been the medical chair for NYC and Long Island Go Red for Women luncheons for many years, working as a national spokesperson to raise awareness about heart disease prevention, diagnosis and treatment opportunities for women.

She currently serves as a member of the Scientific Advisory Council for WomenHeart: The National Coalition for Women with Heart Disease.

Dr. Rosen is a member of the Roundtable on Health Literacy at the National Academy of Medicine (formerly, the Institute of Medicine), where her work focuses on the importance of health literacy tenets and cultural competency initiatives in order to optimize health and wellness for women.

Dr. Rosen served two terms as an American College of Cardiology Councilor, serving Nassau and Suffolk Counties. She has received numerous teaching awards including the Ann Gottlieb Award for Excellence in teaching from Northwell Health-LIJ, and awards for volunteer service from the American Heart Association and was voted one of Long Island's Top 50 Most Influential Women on two occasions. She received the Mets Foundation Every Woman Matters Award and the Cardiovascular Science Award from the American Heart Association at the 48th annual American Heart Ball for the Long Island region.

Dr. Rosen currently lives in Nassau County, New York, with her husband, Dr. Mark Silverman.

SOTIRIA EVERETT, RD, EdD, is a Registered Dietitian Nutritionist and Clinical Assistant Professor in the Department of Family, Population and Preventive Medicine's Nutrition Division at Stony Brook University. Prior to joining Stony Brook University, Dr. Everett was the nutritionist at the Katz Institute for Women's Health at Northwell Health where she created a comprehensive ambulatory nutrition program as part of an integrated health care service.

A graduate of Teachers College, Columbia University, Dr. Everett is also a member of the Academy of Nutrition and Dietetics and a board certified sports dietitian. She has co-authored several chapters for nutrition textbooks and articles for scientific journals. Dr. Everett has also been featured in several media outlets, such as *SHAPE* magazine, *Women's Health* and *Girl's Life* magazine.

LORI M. RUSSO, JD, is a consultant with a focus on women's health. Prior to starting her own consulting business, Ms. Russo was in-house counsel (1986 to 2011) and Americas Head of Employee Recognition and Alumni Relations (2011-2012) for Credit Suisse, a multinational financial services company. Since 2012, Ms. Russo has concentrated on projects related to health care, with a specific focus on women's health and gender disparities. Recent projects include the two-part PBS documentary series *Rx: The Quiet Revolution* and *Rx: Doctors of Tomorrow*. She is a graduate of Northwestern University and the Boston University School of Law.

THE KATZ INSTITUTE FOR WOMEN'S HEALTH AT NORTHWELL HEALTH is dedicated to forging a new model of women's health. KIWH focuses on the unique medical needs of women across their lifespan, by creating a lifelong partnership through the delivery of coordinated sex- and gender-based clinical care, health education targeting prevention and well-being and the support of sex- and gender-specific research.

Index

D

Y

11/22